Natural Healing Handbook

200+ Herbal Remedies for Stress, Better Sleep, Immunity, Digestion, and Everyday Wellness

Gabriel Cress

This book is for educational purposes only and does not replace professional medical advice, diagnosis, or treatment.

When to Seek Medical Care

Stop using natural remedies and consult a healthcare provider immediately if you experience chest pain, difficulty breathing, severe headache, high fever lasting more than 48 hours, unexplained weight loss, persistent vomiting, blood in urine or stool, sudden vision changes, or any symptoms that worsen or don't improve within a reasonable timeframe. Natural remedies should never delay proper medical evaluation for serious conditions.

Safety Considerations

The remedies in this book are generally considered safe for minor, everyday ailments when used as directed. However, individual responses vary significantly. What works well for one person may cause adverse reactions in another. Always start with small amounts to test your tolerance. Pregnant and nursing women, children under 12, elderly adults, and anyone with chronic health conditions or taking prescription medications should consult their healthcare provider before trying any herbal remedy. Many herbs interact with common medications including blood thinners, diabetes medications, blood pressure drugs, and antidepressants.

Limitations and Liability

This book cannot diagnose medical conditions or prescribe treatments. The author is sharing traditional knowledge and personal experience, not providing medical counsel. Natural remedies work best as complementary support alongside conventional medicine, not as replacements for it. By using the information in this book, you acknowledge that you do so at your own risk. Neither the author nor publisher can be held responsible for any adverse effects or consequences resulting from the use of any suggestions, preparations, or procedures described herein.

Remember: When in doubt, always consult a qualified healthcare professional. Your health and safety should always be your primary concern.

Table of Content

About Me and Why I Wrote This Book

I didn't grow up thinking I would one day write about herbs or natural healing. In fact, for a long time I thought those things belonged to another time, something my grandmother knew, but not really useful in a modern life. She was the one who first showed me that a cup of tea or a simple homemade remedy could bring real comfort. As a child, I didn't see the wisdom in it; I just thought it was sweet that she cared enough to make something for me when I wasn't feeling well.

Many years later, during a period of stress and sleepless nights, I found myself lost. I didn't have a grand plan or a perfect solution. I just reached for what I remembered: chamomile, lavender, lemon balm. To my surprise, those small rituals helped. Not in a dramatic, instant way, but in a steady, gentle way that reminded me to slow down and take care of myself.

I wish I could say I figured it all out from there, but the truth is it was messy. Some remedies worked, some didn't. I brewed teas that tasted awful, tried routines I quickly abandoned, and doubted myself more than once. But I kept coming back, curious about why some of these practices seemed to hold a kind of quiet truth. That curiosity led me to read more, to learn from others, and to experiment in my own everyday life.

And when I say "experiment," I mean it quite literally: my kitchen table has often been crowded with jars of dried leaves, scribbled notes, and spoons stained with turmeric. I've overwatered plants on my balcony and forgotten jars of tinctures at the back of the cupboard. Not every attempt was a success, but each one taught me something.

Outside of that, I'm just a fairly ordinary person. I like walking in nature when I can, collecting little sprigs of herbs or simply enjoying the silence of trees after rain. I cook simple meals, read novels on quiet evenings, and sometimes fall asleep with too many books piled on my nightstand. None of this makes me an expert, it just makes me someone who's curious and still learning, just like you.

This book grew out of that mix, memories, trial and error, tradition, and a lot of honest searching. I don't see myself as an authority with all the answers. I'm simply sharing what I've discovered along the way, in the hope that it might bring you the same comfort and support it has brought me.

My hope is simple: that these pages feel like an open door, not a lecture. That you feel free to try, to adapt, to leave behind what doesn't serve you and hold on to what does. And maybe, as you go through these recipes and practices, you'll find your own version of what I once found in my grandmother's kitchen, a sense of comfort, care, and connection that feels both timeless and deeply personal.

Part 1 – The Basics

Everyday life is filled with moments when you pause and wonder how to take care of yourself in the simplest way. A heavy meal leaves you feeling uncomfortable, a long day brings tension to your shoulders, or a restless night makes it hard to think clearly the next morning. These small challenges may not be emergencies, yet they shape the way you feel, think, and move through your day.

This first part of the book is here to give you a foundation. Before exploring the many recipes that follow, it is important to understand what natural healing really means, how it differs from quick fixes, and when it is most useful. These are the basics you can always return to when you feel uncertain or overwhelmed.

In the chapters ahead, you will:

- **Define natural healing:** Learn what it truly is and how simple ingredients like herbs, spices, and kitchen staples can become everyday tools for comfort and support.

- **Recognize different types of care:** Understand the difference between calming a symptom in the moment and supporting your body at a deeper level.

- **Know when to act on your own and when to seek help:** See clear examples of situations where a natural remedy is enough, and where medical guidance is essential.

- **Set the philosophy for the entire book:** Discover the approach that makes these remedies practical, safe, and easy to integrate into modern routines.

The purpose of this section is not to overwhelm you with theory but to offer clarity. Once you know the essentials, everything that follows will feel easier to use. Instead of wondering whether an herbal tea or a simple compress could really make a difference, you will have the confidence to prepare it and notice the results.

Think of this part as your starting point. It gives you the knowledge you need to move forward with certainty, while keeping the focus on practical, everyday solutions. With these basics in place, you will be ready to explore the wide variety of remedies in the next section and use them in a way that makes sense for your life.

What is Natural Healing

It starts with something small. You wake up with a dull headache after a long workday. The to-do list is longer than the hours in your schedule, and your shoulders carry the weight of everything you didn't get done yesterday. You reach for a glass of water, press your fingers gently to your temples, and wonder: *Is there something simple I can do right now to feel better?*

Moments like these are part of everyday life. Stress, tension, indigestion, sleepless nights, they arrive without warning, and often at the least convenient time. You don't always want to reach for a pill, and sometimes you don't even need to. Right in your kitchen, on your windowsill, or in your garden, there are natural tools that can help your body regain balance. That is where natural healing begins: with the practical use of nature's resources to support your health in real time.

Natural healing is the practice of using remedies derived from plants, herbs, and other elements found in nature to support your well-being. It includes herbal teas that soothe your nerves, compresses that calm irritated skin, and simple pantry staples like honey or ginger that ease discomfort. These approaches rely on centuries of traditional knowledge, updated with modern understanding, to provide safe, accessible ways to care for your body.

Think of natural healing as everyday self-care with the help of the earth's ingredients. It doesn't require special equipment or rare products. A sprig of fresh mint, a spoonful of chamomile flowers, a pinch of cinnamon — these are not exotic luxuries but items you might already keep at home. When you prepare them with intention, they become allies for your health.

What makes natural healing valuable is its practicality. It gives you the ability to respond to small challenges, from a restless night to a heavy meal, with gentle, supportive measures. At the same time, it reflects a tradition that has been passed down through generations. People have always turned to plants and natural substances for comfort, and in a modern world filled with constant stimuli, that wisdom has even greater relevance.

Symptom Relief vs. Root Support

When you feel unwell, it's tempting to focus only on stopping the discomfort. For example, if your head is pounding, you might rub a cool cloth across your forehead. The immediate sensation is soothing, and the pain often eases for a while. That is symptom relief — it helps you feel better in the moment.

Root support goes deeper. Instead of just calming a headache, it asks: *Why is my body producing this pain?* Maybe you're dehydrated. Maybe stress has been building all week. Perhaps your sleep has been irregular. In that case, drinking more water throughout the day, taking short breaks to breathe, or adjusting your evening routine addresses the cause rather than just the signal.

Another example is digestive discomfort. A quick solution could be sipping a warm herbal infusion after a heavy meal. It helps temporarily, but if your meals are rushed or consistently too heavy, the same issue will return. Supporting your digestion at its root might mean choosing foods that are easier to process or eating at a slower pace.

Natural healing honors both sides. There are times when you simply need fast comfort, and there are moments when your body is asking for deeper support. Knowing how to combine both gives you flexibility, so you can handle immediate discomfort while also strengthening your overall well-being.

When to Use It and When to Seek Medical Support

Natural remedies are well suited for daily discomforts and minor challenges. You can reach for them when:

- You're feeling stressed or tense after a demanding day.
- A mild cold leaves you with a runny nose and fatigue.
- Your stomach feels heavy or bloated after a meal.
- You want to settle your mind before bedtime.
- You're looking for small boosts of energy without overstimulation.

In these cases, natural healing can be a first response — a way to care for yourself before turning to stronger interventions. A cup of warm tea, a calming bath, or a simple herbal compress can ease your body back toward balance.

There are, however, situations where professional medical help is essential. Severe or persistent pain, unexplained weight changes, chest discomfort, high fever, shortness of breath, or chronic conditions like diabetes or heart disease require professional evaluation. Natural remedies can support your healing, but they cannot replace medical care.

Safety Note

The remedies in this book are designed for everyday use and general wellness. They are not a substitute for medical treatment. If you are pregnant, nursing, taking prescription medication, or dealing with a serious or chronic condition, consult a qualified healthcare professional before trying new remedies.

The Philosophy Behind This Book

Every home can hold a small collection of natural remedies, ready to support you in moments of need. You don't have to wait for a crisis or spend hours studying botany. You can begin with what you already know and what you already have, and expand at your own rhythm.

The purpose of these pages is to make natural healing accessible, safe, and usable in daily life. You'll find practical, straightforward solutions, over 200 of them, organized so you can pick what you need in any moment. The goal is not perfection, but progress: each small step adds up to a healthier, calmer, and more balanced way of living.

Your Natural Healing Toolkit

Y ou open the kitchen cupboard, looking for something to settle your stomach after a heavy dinner. Your eyes pass over a jar of honey, a bag of dried mint, a lemon sitting in a bowl. They seem ordinary at first glance, but each one can become the base of a natural remedy. What feels like clutter on a shelf can quickly turn into a calming tea, a soothing drink, or a simple rub that brings relief.

Starting with natural healing does not require a trip to a distant herb farm or hours of study. The essentials are already around you, waiting to be noticed. This chapter will show you how to build a small collection of herbs, everyday ingredients, and simple tools that you can use immediately. Think of it as creating your first set of building blocks — the foundation for everything that follows.

Everyday Herbs & Ingredients

To begin, it helps to know which plants and foods are the most versatile. Below you'll find a selection of familiar items. Each one has a place in a beginner's kit and can be used in many different ways.

	Chamomile Known for its soft floral flavor, chamomile is often turned into a calming tea before bed. It can ease restlessness and support relaxation.
	Ginger Warming and slightly spicy, ginger is valued for bringing comfort after a heavy meal and for giving a gentle lift of energy when you feel sluggish.
	Mint Fresh and cooling, mint supports digestion and clears the head. A few leaves in hot water or even just crushed in your hands release a refreshing scent.
	Lemon Bright and tangy, lemon can help you feel more awake and refreshed. A slice in water is often enough to lighten a heavy morning.

Honey

Naturally sweet, honey coats the throat and can soften irritation. It also adds flavor and comfort to warm drinks.

Turmeric

Recognized for its golden color, turmeric is used in warm drinks or added to meals to support the body's natural balance.

Cinnamon

This warming spice brings depth to teas and drinks. It can make a simple preparation feel grounding and comforting.

Garlic

A kitchen staple, garlic supports overall vitality. Adding it to meals is one of the easiest ways to bring its benefits into your routine.

Sage

Often used in cooking, sage also supports clarity and comfort. Its leaves can be steeped for a gentle herbal tea.

Lavender

With its distinctive floral aroma, lavender is often used for relaxation. A few dried blossoms are enough to create a soothing scent or a mild infusion.

Rosemary

This herb carries a clean, pine-like fragrance. It can refresh the mind and add a vibrant note to teas or meals.

These ingredients are affordable, easy to find, and endlessly useful. By keeping them at hand, you give yourself a set of natural options you can rely on in daily life.

Simple Tools You Need

You don't need to turn your home into a laboratory. A handful of simple tools is enough to prepare most remedies.

	Mortar and pestle Crush dried herbs or seeds to release their natural compounds.
	Small pot Heat water for teas and infusions without special equipment.
	Glass jars with lids Store dried herbs, infused oils, or homemade blends.
	Strainers or cheesecloth Separate liquid from plant material when preparing teas, broths, or infused oils.
	Measuring spoons Ensure you use consistent amounts.
	Spray bottles Perfect for homemade mists or refreshing blends.
	Clean cotton cloths or gauze Useful for compresses and topical applications.

Most of these items are inexpensive and may already be in your kitchen. As you grow more comfortable, you can add a few extras, but the basics are all you need to start.

Setting Up Your Healing Corner

A small, dedicated space makes it easier to use your remedies regularly. It doesn't have to be a large cabinet or a full pantry. A single shelf, a basket, or even a tray on your kitchen counter can become your herbal corner. Place your jars of herbs where you can see them. Add simple labels with the name and date, so you always know what's fresh. A small box can hold cloths, spoons, and a strainer. If you enjoy creating a calming atmosphere, a candle or a small plant can make the space feel welcoming. Think of this corner as a reminder that you have what you need within reach. Every time you pass by, it invites you to pause, take a breath, and remember that health support can start with something as simple as boiling water and a pinch of herbs.

To make your first steps even easier, keep this quick-start list at hand. It shows what each basic ingredient supports and the fastest way to use it today.

Ingredient	Main Support	Easiest Use
Chamomile	Relaxation, calm	Evening tea
Ginger	Digestive comfort, energy	Slice in hot water
Mint	Freshness, clarity	Add fresh leaves to water
Lemon	Refreshing, digestive support	Squeeze into warm water
Honey	Throat soothing, gentle energy	Stir into tea or warm milk
Turmeric	Natural balance, warmth	Mix with warm milk or tea
Cinnamon	Warming, grounding	Add to tea or oatmeal
Garlic	Vitality, support	Use in cooking
Sage	Clear breathing, digestive support	Brew as tea
Lavender	Calm, gentle relaxation	Add blossoms to bath or tea
Rosemary	Focus, circulation	Brew in hot water or use as rinse

You already have more resources at home than you realize. A jar of herbs, a handful of spices, or a bottle of honey can become the first step toward a new way of caring for yourself. By setting up your own toolkit, you create a space that makes action easier.

From here, the next step is simple: learning how to turn these basic items into remedies you can use whenever you need them. That's what comes next.

How to Prepare & Store Remedies

This chapter is your practical toolbox. Here you'll learn the basic methods that transform herbs and everyday ingredients into remedies you can sip, apply, or store for later. Each technique is simple and approachable. With a few household items and a bit of practice, you'll be able to create your own collection of supportive preparations.

The Main Preparation Techniques

Infusions and Teas

An infusion is one of the easiest ways to draw out the qualities of delicate herbs such as leaves and flowers. You simply cover the plant material with hot water and let it rest. The warmth extracts flavor and supportive compounds into the liquid.

Example:

- Place 1 teaspoon of dried chamomile in a cup.
- Pour hot water over it.
- Cover and wait about 5 minutes before sipping.

Decoctions

Some parts of plants, such as roots and bark, are tougher and need more time. A decoction involves simmering these parts in water so their properties can be released.

Example:

- Add 1 teaspoon of dried ginger root to a small pot with one cup of water.
- Bring to a gentle simmer for 10 minutes.
- Strain and drink warm.

Herbal Oils and Infused Oils

When you soak herbs in oil, the plant's natural components merge with the oil. These infusions are often used for skin support or gentle massage.

Example:

- Place a small handful of dried lavender flowers in a clean jar.
- Cover with olive oil until submerged.
- Let sit in a warm spot for two weeks, then strain into a fresh container.

Salves and Balms

A salve is a thick preparation that sits on the skin, forming a protective layer. It is often made by blending infused oil with a natural wax such as beeswax.

Example:

- Melt 2 tablespoons of infused oil with 1 teaspoon of beeswax.
- Stir until smooth.
- Pour into a small tin and let it cool before using.

Syrups and Gummies

Sweet bases like honey or sugar can hold the qualities of herbs. These are useful for soothing the throat or encouraging hydration.

Example:

- Warm half a cup of honey gently.
- Add a few slices of fresh lemon.
- Let it cool and use a spoonful as needed.

Steams and Inhalations

Breathing in warm, moist air infused with herbs can ease discomfort in your nose and chest.

Example:

- Boil a pot of water and remove it from heat.
- Add a spoonful of dried peppermint leaves.
- Lean over carefully with a towel over your head to breathe in the steam.

Baths and Foot Soaks

Water itself can carry the benefits of herbs into your skin and muscles. Adding simple ingredients to a bath or foot basin can shift your energy after a long day.

Example:

- Fill a bowl with warm water.
- Add a handful of dried sage leaves.
- Soak your feet for fifteen minutes.

Powders and Capsules

Grinding dried herbs into a fine powder allows you to use them in food, drinks, or homemade capsules. This is a practical way to include herbs regularly.

Example:

- Grind dried cinnamon sticks into a fine powder.
- Mix half a teaspoon into your morning oatmeal.
- Store the rest in a small jar.

Storage and Shelf Life

Once you prepare a remedy, storing it properly helps keep it fresh and effective. Clean containers are essential. Glass jars with tight lids prevent air and moisture from reducing the quality of dried herbs. For infused oils or syrups, use sterilized bottles and keep them away from direct sunlight. A cupboard that stays cool and dark is often the best choice.

Label each container with the name of the herb or preparation and the date you made it. This small step saves you from guessing later. As a general guide:

- **Dried herbs** stay fresh for about 6 to 12 months when sealed and stored away from heat and light.
- **Infused oils** are best used within 2 to 3 months unless kept in the refrigerator.
- **Herbal syrups** last about 2 to 4 weeks in the fridge, especially those made with honey.
- **Salves and balms** can often last up to 6 months if stored in a clean, airtight container.

These timeframes are guides, not rules. Use your senses. If something changes in color, smell, or texture, it is best to prepare a fresh batch.

Safety

Respecting dosage and quality is essential. A small amount of an herb may be comforting, while too much can cause discomfort. Start with modest portions and notice how your body responds.

Pay attention to any unusual reactions such as itching, rashes, or stomach upset. If that happens, stop using the remedy and consider speaking with a health professional.

Some herbs interact with medications or may not be recommended during pregnancy or for people with specific conditions. Whenever you feel unsure, seek professional advice before trying something new. Listening to your body and asking for guidance when necessary is part of caring for yourself wisely.

Part 2 – Practical Remedies for Everyday Life

O nce you know the basics, the next step is action. Knowledge is useful, but it only becomes meaningful when you can apply it in your daily routine. This section has been designed as a practical collection of recipes that you can consult at any moment. Each page is clear, concise, and focused on one specific need, so you do not have to search long to find what helps.

Instead of reading this section from start to finish, you can use it like a reference shelf. Open it whenever you face a small discomfort or want to support your body in a simple way. The remedies are organized by theme, which makes it easy to navigate: stress and focus, better sleep, immunity, digestion, hormonal balance, skin and hair care, relief for muscles, and quick first aid.

Here is how to approach this part of the book:

- **Identify your need:** Look at the table of contents and go directly to the section that matches your current situation, whether it is tension, a headache, or a heavy stomach.

- **Choose a form that fits your moment:** Teas and infusions are ideal when you have a few minutes to pause. Sprays and inhalers work well on the go. Baths, soaks, or compresses are best for evenings or when you can dedicate a little more time.

- **Keep it simple:** Most recipes require only two or three ingredients and basic kitchen tools such as a pot, a jar, or a spoon. You do not need to invest in special equipment to benefit.

- **Use what you have:** Many of the herbs and foods included are common and often already at home. A lemon, some mint, or a spoonful of honey can become a quick remedy with almost no effort.

- **Think of consistency, not perfection:** You do not need to prepare every recipe. Even using one or two regularly can provide noticeable support.

The strength of this section lies in its practicality. Every recipe is presented in the same format so you can quickly understand what it is for, what you need, and how to prepare it. There is no long theory here, only direct applications.

From the next page onward, you will step into a catalog of more than two hundred remedies. They are grouped by purpose, so you can easily find the right support at the right time. Keep this part close and treat it as your personal toolbox for everyday wellness.

Stress, Focus & Mental Energy

Stress, distraction, and mental fatigue are challenges most people face on a daily basis. You sit down to get something done, but your mind drifts between emails, messages, and unfinished tasks. By midday you may feel drained, tense in your shoulders, or restless in your thoughts. Many people turn to another cup of coffee or a sugary snack to push through, but those quick fixes often bring short bursts of energy followed by an even sharper crash.

The remedies in this chapter are designed to offer a different kind of support: practical, natural, and easy to prepare. You don't need special tools or exotic ingredients. A handful of herbs, a slice of lemon, a spoonful of honey, or a sprig of mint can become effective allies in restoring calm and clarity.

The recipes ahead are grouped by purpose to make your choice simple:

- **Calming teas and infusions** that help release tension and quiet the nervous system when stress runs high.

- **Energizing tonics and drinks** that stimulate circulation and lift your mood without overstimulation.

- **Aromatic sprays and inhalations** that provide quick, portable ways to refresh your focus when you feel distracted or mentally heavy.

These preparations fit into the rhythm of everyday life. You might use a morning tonic instead of reaching for another espresso, keeping your energy stable as the day begins. During work, a refreshing spray or a pocket inhaler can help you reset your attention between tasks. And in the evening, a warm herbal tea becomes a tool to let go of accumulated stress, allowing your mind and body to prepare for rest.

Each page will give you exactly what you need: a short explanation of when to use the remedy, a clear list of ingredients, and simple steps to follow. Whether you are at home, at the office, or traveling, you'll find options that are quick to prepare and easy to integrate into your daily routine.

With these recipes, managing stress and boosting focus doesn't have to be complicated. You'll learn how to support your mental energy in natural ways, creating small, reliable habits that keep you centered and productive.

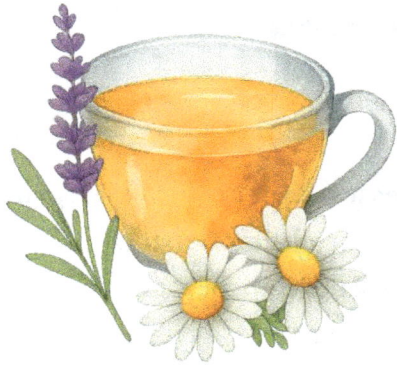

Lavender–Chamomile Evening Tea

A gentle herbal tea that calms the nervous system and eases tension after a long day. Drink in the evening to prepare your body and mind for a restful night.

Ingredients	Instructions
• 1 tsp dried lavender flowers • 1 tsp dried chamomile flowers • 1 cup hot water	1. Place the lavender and chamomile in a mug. 2. Pour hot water over the herbs. 3. Cover and steep for 7 minutes, then strain and sip slowly.

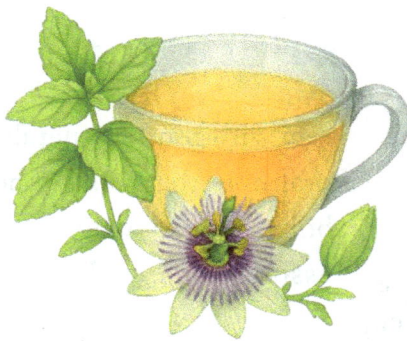

Lemon Balm & Passionflower Tea

This soothing tea eases mental agitation and supports a peaceful state of mind, especially when stress feels overwhelming.

Safety: Avoid passionflower if you are pregnant or taking sedatives without medical guidance.

Ingredients	Instructions
• 1 tsp dried lemon balm leaves • 1 tsp dried passionflower • 1 cup hot water	1. Combine the herbs in a cup. 2. Pour hot water over them. 3. Cover and let steep for 8–10 minutes. Strain before drinking.

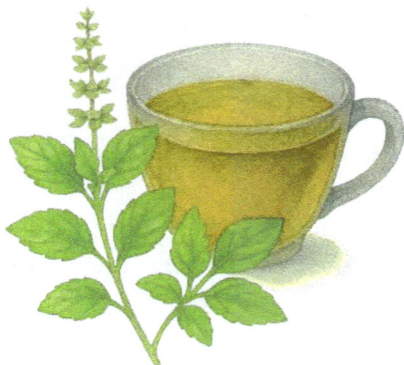

Holy Basil Stress-Relief Infusion

Tulsi, or holy basil, has been treasured for centuries as a gentle adaptogen that restores balance after emotional or physical stress. Its warm, slightly peppery taste encourages a sense of calm and helps clear the mental fog of long days. Enjoy this infusion as a daily reset ritual.

Ingredients	Instructions
• 1 tbsp dried holy basil leaves • 1 tsp honey (optional) • 1 cup hot water	1. Place holy basil in a mug. 2. Pour hot water and cover for 5–7 minutes. 3. Strain, add honey if desired, and sip slowly.

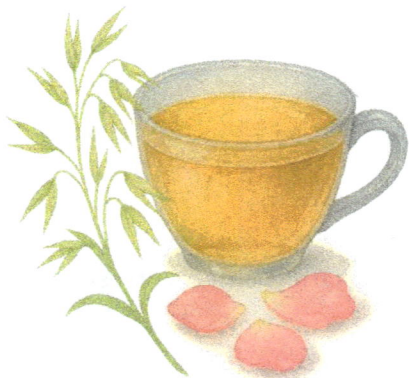

Oatstraw & RosePetal Tea

Oatstraw nourishes the nervous system with gentle minerals, while rose petals add a soothing floral note that uplifts the spirit. Together they help ease irritability, soften tension, and bring emotional comfort during stressful moments. This tea feels like a warm embrace in a cup.

Ingredients	Instructions
• 1 tbsp dried oatstraw • 1 tsp dried rose petals • 1 cup hot water	1. Place oatstraw and rose petals in a teapot or mug. 2. Add hot water and cover. 3. Let steep for 10 minutes, then strain before drinking.

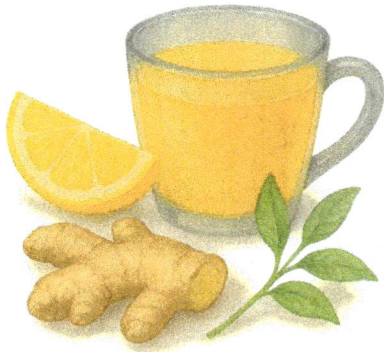

Ginger–Lemon Morning Tonic

This bright, invigorating tonic wakes up your senses and prepares you for the day ahead. Ginger's warming spice stimulates circulation and boosts vitality, while lemon adds freshness that sharpens focus and lifts your mood.

Tip: Drink on an empty stomach for a gentle energy boost without jitters.

Ingredients	Instructions
• 1 tsp fresh grated ginger • 1 slice fresh lemon • 1 cup hot water	1. Place ginger in a mug and pour hot water over it. 2. Steep for 5 minutes. 3. Add the lemon slice and enjoy warm.

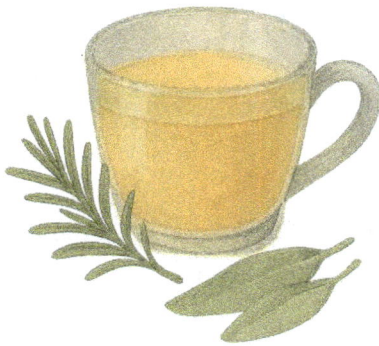

Rosemary & Sage Focus Tea

Aromatic and earthy, this tea is ideal when you need mental clarity and sharper memory. Rosemary awakens the mind with its refreshing scent, while sage provides a grounding effect that helps you concentrate on tasks. Perfect for study sessions or focused work.

Ingredients	Instructions
• 1 tsp dried rosemary • 1 tsp dried sage • 1 cup hot water	1. Combine rosemary and sage in a teapot. 2. Pour hot water and cover. 3. Steep for 6–8 minutes, then strain before drinking.

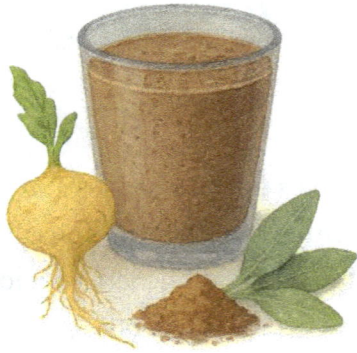

Maca–Cacao Vitality Smoothie

This creamy smoothie blends the earthy depth of maca with the rich flavor of raw cacao, creating a nourishing energy lift. It fuels both body and mind, helping you stay motivated without the crash that often follows coffee or energy drinks. Enjoy it as a mid-morning or afternoon pick-me-up.

Ingredients	Instructions
• 1 cup milk or plant-based milk • 1 tsp maca powder • 1 tsp raw cacao powder • 1 tsp honey (optional)	1. Place all ingredients in a blender. 2. Blend until smooth and frothy. 3. Pour into a glass and drink slowly.

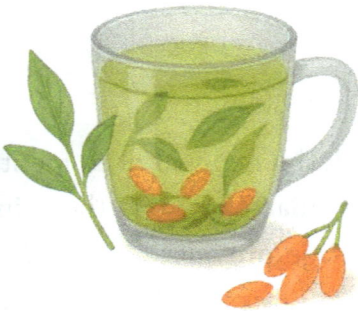

Green Tea & Goji Berry Infusion

A gentle infusion that combines the clean lift of green tea with the natural sweetness and antioxidants of goji berries. It provides steady energy without overstimulation, while supporting your overall vitality. Delicious served hot or chilled, making it versatile for any time of day.

Ingredients	Instructions
• 1 tsp green tea leaves • 1 tbsp dried goji berries • 1 cup hot water	1. Place green tea and goji berries in a mug. 2. Pour hot water and cover. 3. Steep for 5 minutes, then strain and sip.

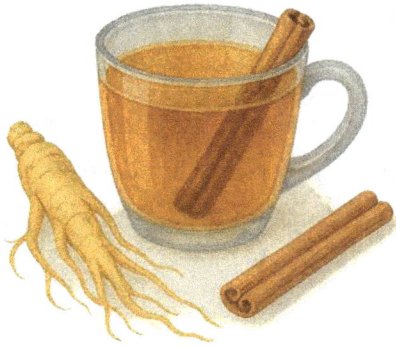

Ginseng & Cinnamon Energy Brew

This warming brew combines ginseng's reputation for enhancing stamina with cinnamon's naturally uplifting spice. It can help you push through long afternoons or add motivation when energy dips. A balanced way to recharge without relying on heavy stimulants.

Ingredients	Instructions
• 1 tsp dried ginseng root slices • 1 small cinnamon stick • 1 cup water	1. Place ginseng and cinnamon in a small pot with water. 2. Bring to a gentle simmer for 10 minutes. 3. Strain and enjoy warm.

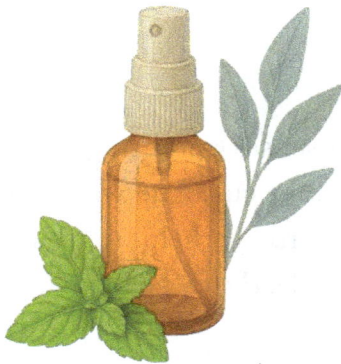

Peppermint & Eucalyptus Focus Spray

A crisp, cooling mist that instantly refreshes the senses when fatigue sets in. Peppermint sharpens attention, while eucalyptus clears mental heaviness, making it perfect for your desk, study space, or even a midday reset.

Safety: Do not spray directly on skin or eyes; keep out of children's reach.

Ingredients	Instructions
• ½ cup distilled water • 5 drops peppermint essential oil • 3 drops eucalyptus essential oil	1. Pour water into a clean spray bottle. 2. Add the essential oils and shake well. 3. Mist lightly in the air around you.

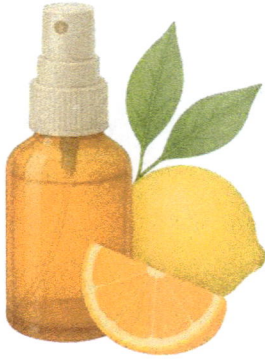

Citrus Uplift Room Mist

This bright and cheerful mist helps energize any indoor space with its lively aroma. The blend of orange and lemon essential oils can lighten the atmosphere, improve mood, and give you a gentle push when your motivation feels low.

Ingredients	Instructions
• ½ cup distilled water • 5 drops sweet orange essential oil • 3 drops lemon essential oil	1. Pour water into a spray bottle. 2. Add the essential oils. 3. Shake before each use and spritz into the air.

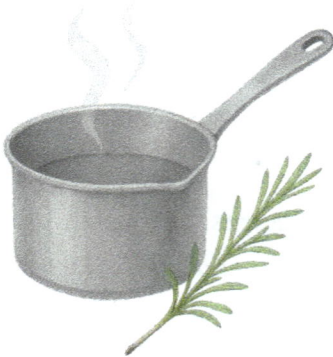

Rosemary Steam for Mental Clarity

A fragrant steam that clears the senses and brings sharper focus during moments of mental fatigue. The warm vapor carries the herb's invigorating aroma, helping you feel refreshed and ready to think more clearly.

Ingredients	Instructions
• 2 tsp dried rosemary • 3 cups hot water	1. Place rosemary in a large bowl. 2. Pour hot water over it. 3. Lean over with a towel over your head and inhale deeply for 5–10 minutes.

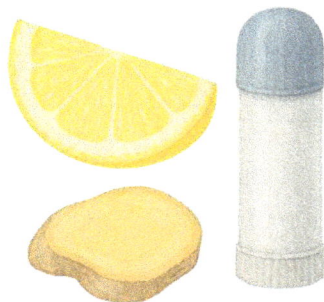

Lemon–Ginger Pocket Inhaler

This handy inhaler offers quick relief when your energy dips or your mind feels foggy. The bright citrus and warming spice create an instant lift, making it easy to carry mental clarity wherever you go.

Ingredients	Instructions
• 5 drops lemon essential oil • 3 drops ginger essential oil • 1 cotton wick or pad • 1 small inhaler tube or vial with lid	1. Insert the cotton wick into the inhaler tube. 2. Add essential oils onto the wick. 3. Inhale through the tube whenever you need a burst of focus.

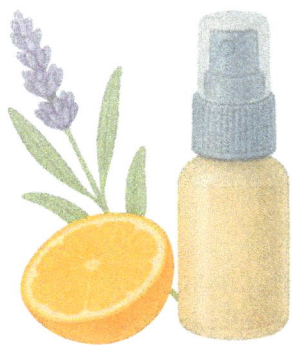

Stress-Relief Desk Spray (Lavender & Orange)

A gentle aromatic spray that soothes tension and restores a sense of calm while you work. Lavender relaxes the nervous system, while sweet orange brightens the mood, creating a balanced atmosphere at your desk.

Ingredients	Instructions
• ½ cup distilled water • 4 drops lavender essential oil • 4 drops sweet orange essential oil	1. Pour water into a spray bottle. 2. Add the essential oils. 3. Shake gently and mist around your workspace.

Better Sleep Naturally

A good night's sleep is one of the strongest foundations for overall well-being, yet it is often the first thing we sacrifice when life gets busy. Late-night screen time, unfinished tasks, or a racing mind can keep you awake long past the moment you intended to rest. Over time, those lost hours add up, leaving you tired in the morning, foggy during the day, and more sensitive to stress.

The remedies in this chapter are designed to support your natural ability to wind down and rest. They focus on making bedtime calmer, your body more relaxed, and your mind ready to let go of the day. Instead of relying on heavy sleep aids, you can create simple, gentle preparations that encourage your body to follow its natural rhythm.

Here's what you'll find in the following pages:

- **Evening teas and infusions** that soothe tension and signal to your body that it's time to slow down. A warm cup of chamomile or valerian root tea can become a nightly ritual that prepares you for deeper sleep.

- **Comforting warm drinks** like golden milk or nutmeg-spiced almond milk, which combine nourishment with relaxation, helping you release the day's stress before bed.

- **Baths and soaks** that use ingredients such as lavender, rose, or Epsom salt to relax tight muscles and create a calming atmosphere for rest.

- **Simple nighttime aids** like pillow sprays, herbal sleep pillows, or gummies that gently release calming aromas or flavors while you drift off.

Most of these remedies require little more than a kettle, a small jar, or a cloth. You can prepare them in minutes, which makes them easy to use even on evenings when you feel too tired to do much. The key is consistency: turning one or two of these practices into regular habits helps your body recognize when it's time to rest.

In the pages ahead, you'll find practical recipes that can be adapted to your lifestyle. Some are perfect for weeknights when you want something quick, while others can become part of a more intentional evening routine. By experimenting with these remedies, you can discover what works best for you and create a bedtime rhythm that truly supports restorative, refreshing sleep.

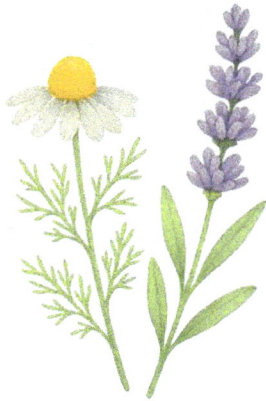

Chamomile–Lavender Bedtime Tea

A calming tea with chamomile and lavender that soothes the mind and eases the body into rest. Drink one cup about 30 minutes before bedtime.

Ingredients	Instructions
<ul><li>1 tsp dried chamomile flowers</li><li>1 tsp dried lavender flowers</li><li>1 cup hot water</li></ul>	1. Place chamomile and lavender in a mug. 2. Pour hot water over the herbs. 3. Cover and steep for 7 minutes, then strain and sip slowly. *Tip: Covering the cup preserves calming aromas.*

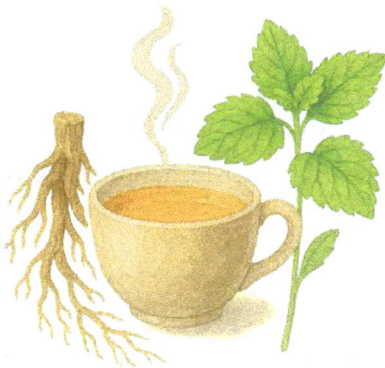

Valerian Root & Lemon Balm Infusion

This earthy infusion relaxes the nervous system and encourages deep, restorative sleep. Best enjoyed in the late evening. **Safety**: *Avoid valerian if taking sedatives.*

Ingredients	Instructions
<ul><li>1 tsp dried valerian root</li><li>1 tsp dried lemon balm leaves</li><li>1 cup hot water</li></ul>	4. Add valerian root and lemon balm to a teapot. 5. Pour hot water and cover. 6. Steep for 10 minutes, then strain before drinking.

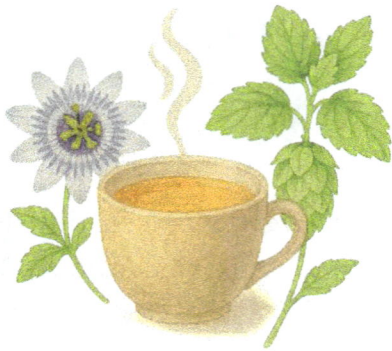

Passionflower & Hops Night Tea

Passionflower and hops reduce nighttime restlessness and support continuous sleep. A gentle night ally when the mind won't quiet down.

Ingredients	Instructions
• 1 tsp dried passionflower • 1 tsp dried hops flowers • 1 cup hot water	1. Place passionflower and hops in a cup. 2. Pour hot water over them. 3. Cover, steep for 8 minutes, then strain.

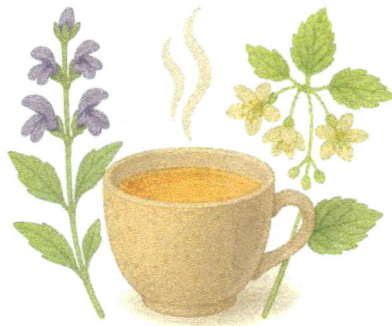

Skullcap & Linden Blossom Infusion

A soothing blend that eases tension and gently calms the nervous system. Ideal before evening routines to prepare for rest.

Ingredients	Instructions
• 1 tsp dried skullcap leaves • 1 tsp dried linden blossoms • 1 cup hot water	1. Add skullcap and linden blossoms to a mug. 2. Pour hot water and cover. 3. Steep for 7–8 minutes, strain, and enjoy.

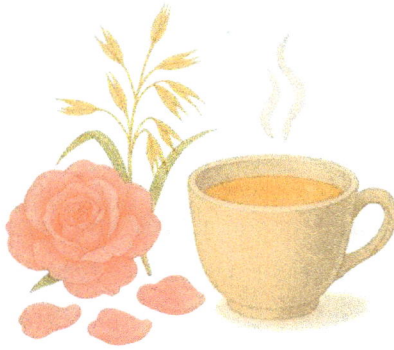

Rose & Oatstraw Evening Tea

Rose petals and oatstraw create a nourishing blend that comforts the senses and guides the body toward peaceful sleep. Drink warm before bed.

Ingredients	Instructions
• 1 tbsp dried oatstraw • 1 tsp dried rose petals • 1 cup hot water	1. Place oatstraw and rose petals in a teapot. 2. Pour hot water, cover, and steep for 10 minutes. 3. Strain before drinking.

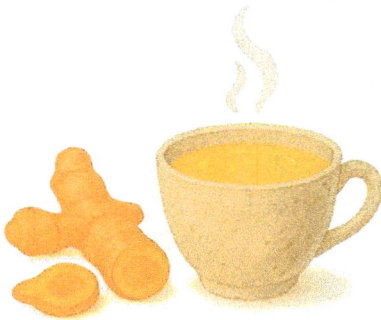

Golden Turmeric Night Milk

This warm golden milk relaxes muscles and eases the body into sleep. A cozy drink that also supports natural balance.

Ingredients	Instructions
• 1 cup warm milk or plant-based milk • ½ tsp turmeric powder • 1 pinch black pepper • 1 tsp honey (optional)	1. Warm the milk gently in a pot. 2. Stir in turmeric and black pepper. 3. Add honey if desired, sip slowly before bed.

Nutmeg & Warm Almond Milk

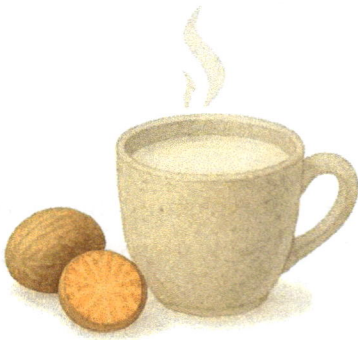

A creamy evening drink that comforts the senses and gently signals the body to release tension. Best enjoyed after evening routines. *Safety: Avoid excess nutmeg, as high doses may cause discomfort.*

Ingredients	Instructions
• 1 cup warm almond milk • ¼ tsp grated nutmeg • 1 tsp honey (optional)	1. Heat almond milk in a small pot. 2. Stir in nutmeg and honey. 3. Drink warm just before bed.

Cocoa–Chamomile Night Drink

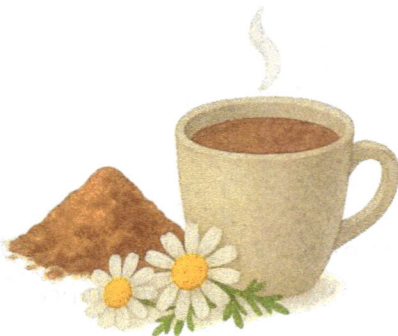

A blend of cocoa's gentle comfort with chamomile's calm for a soothing bedtime ritual. Perfect for those who crave chocolate at night.

Ingredients	Instructions
• 1 cup warm milk or plant-based milk • 1 tsp unsweetened cocoa powder • 1 tsp dried chamomile flowers • 1 tsp honey (optional)	1. Warm the milk in a pot. 2. Add chamomile and steep for 5 minutes. 3. Strain, stir in cocoa and honey, and sip warm.

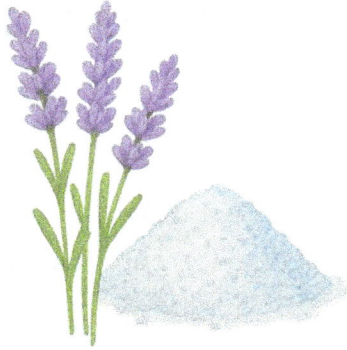

Lavender & Epsom Salt Bath

A relaxing bath that melts away stress and soothes tired muscles. Lavender's aroma supports a calm transition to sleep.

Ingredients	Instructions
• ½ cup dried lavender flowers • 1 cup Epsom salt	1. Mix lavender and Epsom salt in a bowl. 2. Add the blend to warm bathwater. 3. Soak for 20 minutes before bed.

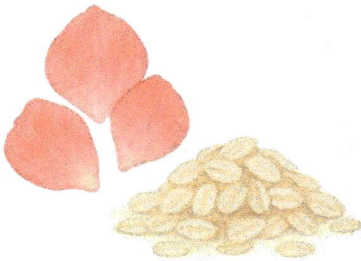

Rose & Oat Bath Soak

Rose and oat combine to soften skin and calm the mind. A gentle soak to prepare body and spirit for nighttime rest.

Ingredients	Instructions
• ½ cup dried rose petals • ½ cup rolled oats (in a muslin bag)	1. Place rose petals and oats into warm bathwater. 2. Let steep for 5 minutes. 3. Soak and relax for 15–20 minutes.

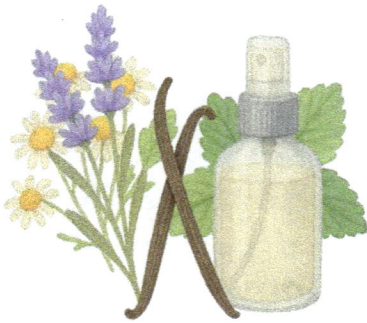

Foot Soak with Chamomile & Lemon Balm

A calming foot soak that eases tension after a long day. Chamomile and lemon balm refresh tired feet and soothe the nervous system.

Ingredients	Instructions
• 2 tbsp dried chamomile flowers • 2 tbsp dried lemon balm leaves • Basin of warm water	1. Place chamomile and lemon balm in the basin. 2. Pour warm water over the herbs. 3. Soak feet for 15–20 minutes before bed.

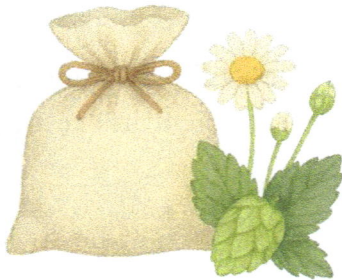

Herbal Sleep Pillow (Chamomile & Hops)

A fragrant sleep pillow filled with chamomile and hops that gently releases relaxing aromas overnight. Place near your head for serene sleep.

Ingredients	Instructions
• ½ cup dried chamomile flowers • ½ cup dried hops flowers • Small cotton or linen pillowcase	1. Fill the pillowcase with chamomile and hops. 2. Sew or tie it shut securely. 3. Place inside or near your pillow at night.

Bedtime Pillow Spray (Lavender & Vanilla)

A soothing pillow spray with lavender and vanilla that creates a calm, inviting bedroom atmosphere. Mist lightly on bedding before sleep.

Ingredients	Instructions
• ½ cup distilled water • 5 drops lavender essential oil • 2 drops vanilla extract or essential oil	1. Pour water into a spray bottle. 2. Add lavender and vanilla. 3. Shake gently before each use and mist onto pillow.

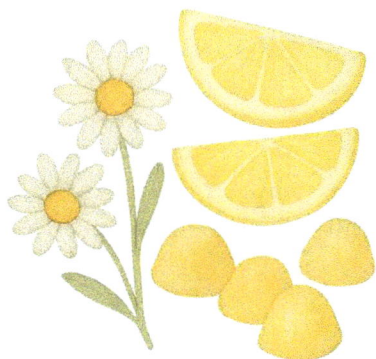

Soothing Sleep Gummies (Chamomile & Lemon)

These gentle gummies combine chamomile and lemon for a sweet, calming bedtime treat. Perfect for adults or children as a nighttime ritual. **Safety:** *Store in the fridge and consume within one week.*

Ingredients	Instructions
• 1 cup chamomile tea (strong brew) • 2 tbsp lemon juice • 2 tbsp honey • 2 tbsp gelatin powder	7. Brew chamomile tea and let it cool slightly. 8. Stir in lemon juice, honey, and gelatin. 9. Pour into silicone molds and refrigerate until set.

Immune Boost & Cold/Flu Support

E veryday health challenges often show up when your body feels most vulnerable, a sudden chill on a damp morning, the first tickle in your throat, or that drained feeling that lingers after a long week. The immune system is your natural defense, but stress, poor sleep, and seasonal changes can make it less resilient. Supporting it doesn't always mean reaching for supplements or over-the-counter pills. Sometimes, the most effective tools are already in your kitchen or garden.

This chapter focuses on natural remedies that strengthen your defenses and bring comfort during cold and flu season. The recipes are grouped into practical categories so you can quickly find what you need:

- **Preventive teas and infusions**: Gentle blends with herbs like echinacea, nettle, or rosehip to nourish your system and help it stay strong during seasonal changes.

- **Tonics and syrups**: Concentrated preparations that combine herbs, spices, and honey to soothe the throat, boost energy, and keep your body prepared for colder months.

- **Quick-response remedies**: Steams, gargles, and lozenges you can use at the first signs of congestion, sore throat, or fatigue.

Most of these remedies are straightforward: a simmered root, a spoonful of honey, or a handful of herbs steeped in hot water. They are designed for convenience, so you can prepare them even when you're not feeling your best. A simple steam can clear your nose before bedtime, while a warm infusion can ease shivers and bring comfort to your chest.

The goal here is not to create complicated routines but to give you reliable, accessible options that fit into daily life. By keeping a few ingredients, like ginger, thyme, or elderberries, on hand, you'll always have a natural way to respond to early symptoms or to maintain strength when everyone around you seems to be catching something.

The following recipes are practical, soothing, and supportive. Use them to stay balanced through the colder months, or turn to them when you feel the first signs of seasonal discomfort. They're small, comforting steps that help you feel more at ease while your body does the work of healing.

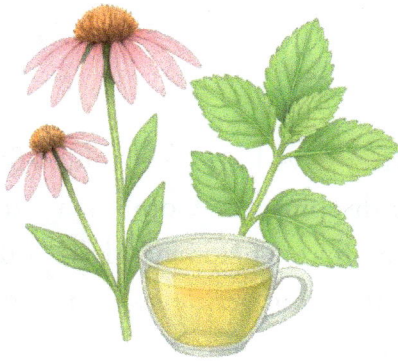

Echinacea & Lemon Balm Tea

This tea blends echinacea's immune-supporting qualities with the gentle calm of lemon balm. It helps the body stay resilient during the colder months while soothing tension often linked to seasonal changes. A cup in the morning can be a comforting daily ritual of protection.

Ingredients	Instructions
• 1 tsp dried echinacea root or leaves • 1 tsp dried lemon balm leaves • 1 cup hot water	1. Place echinacea and lemon balm in a cup. 2. Pour hot water over the herbs. 3. Cover, steep 8–10 minutes, strain, and drink warm.

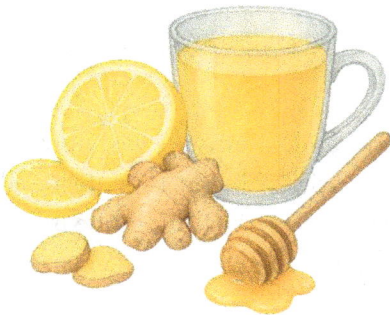

Ginger–Lemon–Honey Infusion

A classic warming blend that comforts the throat, boosts circulation, and provides natural antimicrobial support. The ginger warms from within, lemon refreshes, and honey coats the throat with soothing sweetness. Drink it at the first signs of a cold or after being out in damp weather.

Ingredients	Instructions
• 1 tsp fresh grated ginger • 1 slice fresh lemon • 1 tsp raw honey • 1 cup hot water	1. Add ginger and lemon to a cup. 2. Pour hot water and steep 5 minutes. 3. Strain if desired, stir in honey, and sip warm.

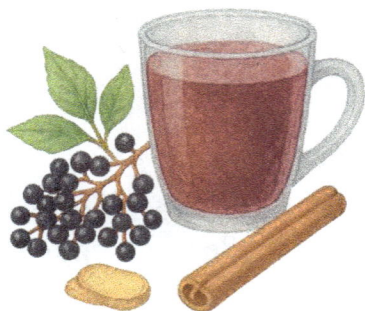

Elderberry & Cinnamon Tea

Rich in antioxidants, elderberries have long been valued for their role in fighting seasonal discomforts. Combined with the warming spice of cinnamon, this tea helps shield the body from colds while bringing comfort and gentle sweetness on cold days.

Ingredients	Instructions
<ul><li>1 tbsp dried elderberries</li><li>1 small cinnamon stick</li><li>1 cup water</li></ul>	1. Simmer elderberries and cinnamon in water for 10 minutes. 2. Remove from heat, cover for 5 minutes. 3. Strain and drink warm.

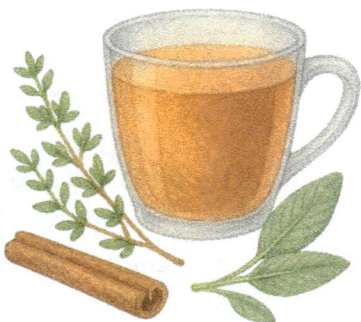

Thyme & Sage Immune Tea

This aromatic tea supports the throat and respiratory system while providing a sense of warmth and clarity. Thyme is traditionally used for clear breathing, while sage soothes irritation in the mouth and throat. Perfect to sip slowly on chilly evenings.

Ingredients	Instructions
<ul><li>1 tsp dried thyme</li><li>1 tsp dried sage leaves</li><li>1 cup hot water</li></ul>	1. Place thyme and sage in a cup. 2. Pour hot water and cover. 3. Steep 7 minutes, strain, and sip slowly.

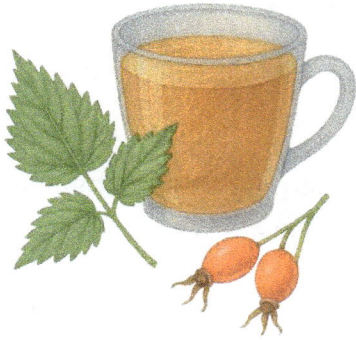

Nettle & Rosehip Infusion

This mineral-rich blend provides a natural source of vitamin C and iron, helping to keep energy levels steady and defenses strong. Its mild, earthy flavor is balanced by the tart brightness of rosehip, making it a nourishing daily tonic throughout fall and winter.

Ingredients	Instructions
<ul><li>1 tbsp dried nettle leaves</li><li>1 tbsp dried rosehips (crushed)</li><li>1 cup hot water</li></ul>	1. Place nettle and rosehips in a teapot. 2. Pour hot water and steep 10 minutes. 3. Strain and enjoy warm or cooled.

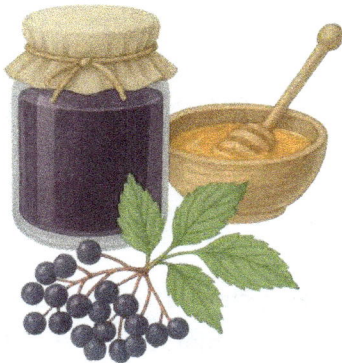

Elderberry Immune Syrup with Honey

A rich, dark syrup that combines elderberries' antiviral support with honey's soothing sweetness. Ideal for children and adults alike, it can be taken daily as prevention or in larger amounts when illness begins. Store in the fridge and keep ready for the season.

Ingredients	Instructions
<ul><li>1 tsp dried thyme</li><li>1 tsp dried sage leaves</li><li>1 cup hot water</li></ul>	1. Place thyme and sage in a cup. 2. Pour hot water and cover. 3. Steep 7 minutes, strain, and sip slowly.

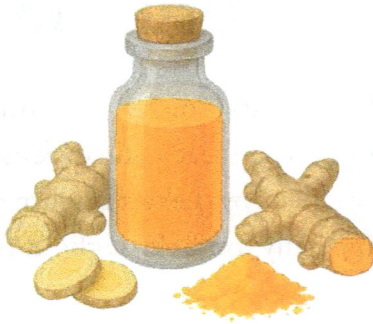

Ginger–Turmeric Immunity Shot

A small but powerful drink that fights seasonal fatigue while supporting the body's natural defenses. Ginger stimulates warmth and circulation, while turmeric provides an anti-inflammatory boost. Take it in the morning when you need quick reinforcement.

Ingredients	Instructions
• 1 inch fresh ginger root, grated • ½ tsp turmeric powder (or fresh grated turmeric) • Juice of ½ lemon • ½ cup water	1. Blend ginger, turmeric, lemon juice, and water. 2. Strain if desired. 3. Drink immediately as a shot.

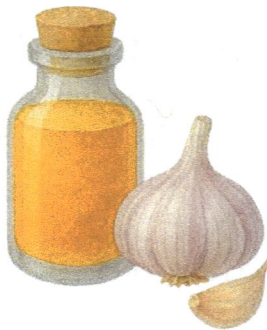

Garlic & Honey Tonic

Garlic has been celebrated for centuries as a natural shield against colds, and honey makes it more palatable while adding its own soothing benefits. This tonic is easy to keep on hand and can be taken by the spoonful each morning to reinforce your immunity.

Ingredients	Instructions
• 5 garlic cloves, peeled and crushed • ½ cup raw honey	1. Place garlic in a clean jar. 2. Cover with honey and stir well. 3. Let infuse 24 hours before use.

Astragalus Root Decoction

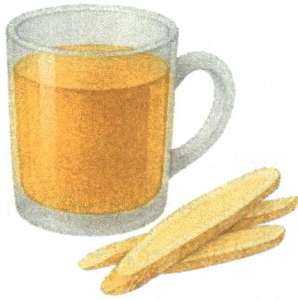

Astragalus root is a classic adaptogen used in traditional Chinese medicine to sustain energy and fortify defenses over time. This gentle decoction is not for acute illness, but for building resilience when taken consistently across the season.

Citrus & Clove Warming

Ingredients	Instructions
• 1 tbsp dried astragalus root slices • 2 cups water	1. Place astragalus in a pot with water. 2. Simmer gently for 20–30 minutes. 3. Strain and sip warm.

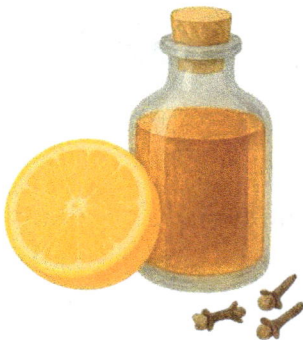

Syrup

This fragrant syrup warms the body from within while easing throat irritation. Orange zest brings brightness and vitamin C, while cloves lend a comforting spice. Take by the spoon on cold evenings or stir into hot water for a warming drink.

Ingredients	Instructions
• Zest of 1 orange • 3 whole cloves • 1 cup water • ½ cup honey	1. Simmer orange zest and cloves in water 10 minutes. 2. Strain and cool slightly. 3. Stir in honey and store in a glass jar.

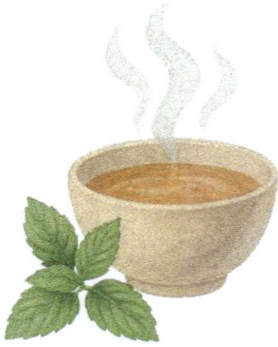

Peppermint Steam for Congestion Relief

A classic steam inhalation that clears nasal passages, refreshes the head, and makes breathing easier. The menthol-rich vapor loosens congestion and helps you feel lighter almost instantly. Use it before bed to ease nighttime breathing.

Ingredients	Instructions
• 2 tbsp dried peppermint leaves • 3 cups hot water	1. Place peppermint in a large bowl. 2. Pour hot water and lean over carefully with a towel. 3. Inhale the steam for 5–10 minutes.

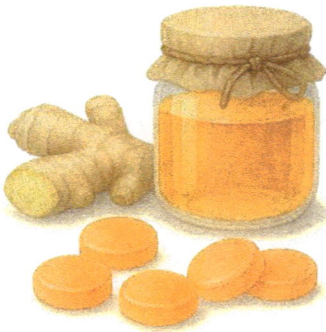

Honey–Ginger Cough Lozenges

These homemade lozenges combine honey's soothing coat with ginger's warming relief, helping to calm coughs and throat irritation. They are easy to carry and provide comfort throughout the day when coughing won't stop.

Ingredients	Instructions
• ½ cup honey • 2 tbsp fresh ginger juice • ½ cup sugar (optional, for texture)	1. Warm honey and ginger juice in a saucepan. 2. Simmer until thickened and sticky. 3. Drop small spoonfuls onto parchment to harden.

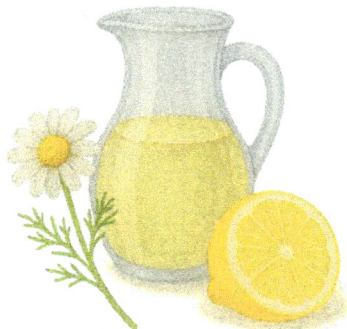

Chamomile & Lemon Gargle

A gentle gargle that calms sore throats and reduces irritation after long days of talking or seasonal strain. Chamomile brings its soothing effect, while lemon adds freshness and mild antibacterial support.

Ingredients	Instructions
<ul><li>1 tsp dried chamomile flowers</li><li>Juice of ½ lemon</li><li>1 cup hot water</li></ul>	1. Brew chamomile tea in hot water, steep 7 minutes. 2. Strain and let cool slightly. 3. Add lemon juice and gargle for 30 seconds.

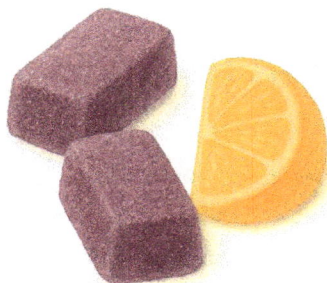

Immune-Boosting Herbal Gummies (Elderberry & Vitamin C)

These soft, sweet gummies are loved by both children and adults. Elderberry provides deep seasonal support, while rosehip offers a natural source of vitamin C. A tasty way to make immunity care part of the daily routine.

Ingredients	Instructions
<ul><li>½ cup honey</li><li>2 tbsp fresh ginger juice</li><li>½ cup sugar (optional, for texture)</li></ul>	1. Warm honey and ginger juice in a saucepan. 2. Simmer until thickened and sticky. 3. Drop small spoonfuls onto parchment to harden.

Gut Health, Digestion & Bloating Relief

D igestive comfort has a direct impact on how you feel throughout the day. When your stomach feels heavy, when bloating makes you uncomfortable, or when irregular digestion slows you down, even the simplest tasks become more difficult. Many people are quick to mask the discomfort with antacids or strong remedies, but your body often needs something gentler that works in harmony with its natural rhythm.

This chapter is designed to give you practical, natural solutions that ease everyday digestive issues and support a healthier gut. The remedies are organized into clear categories so you can find what works best for your needs:

- **Digestive teas and infusions**: Light blends that calm cramping, reduce bloating, and support smoother digestion after meals.

- **Decoctions, broths, and tonics**: More grounding preparations that gently stimulate digestive fire, support the liver, and provide nourishment to the whole body.

- **Practical everyday remedies**: Quick options like chews, sprays, and smoothies that you can use at home or on the go whenever discomfort arises.

These recipes use simple, accessible ingredients such as mint, fennel, ginger, anise, or parsley. They are easy to prepare with common kitchen tools like a mug, a small pot, or a blender. Some can be ready in just a few minutes, making them a convenient first step when you need relief without complicating your day.

Digestive health is not only about solving problems after they appear. It is also about supporting your body consistently, so that meals feel lighter and energy remains steady. A daily tea, a refreshing herbal water, or a warming tonic can become small habits that keep your system balanced over time.

As you explore the following recipes, choose them based on the moment. A gentle tea can ease bloating after dinner. A broth can support you when your stomach feels tired. A quick chew can help during travel or after a heavy meal. Each preparation is designed to be both practical and soothing, giving you a reliable way to care for your digestion whenever you need it.

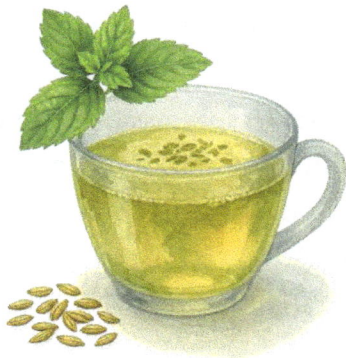

Peppermint & Fennel Digestive Tea

A light, aromatic tea that relieves post-meal bloating and supports smooth digestion. The cooling notes of peppermint ease discomfort, while fennel seeds gently calm gas and support a comfortable stomach after heavy or irregular meals.

Ingredients	Instructions
<ul><li>1 tsp dried peppermint leaves</li><li>1 tsp fennel seeds (lightly crushed)</li><li>1 cup hot water</li></ul>	1. Place the peppermint leaves and crushed fennel seeds in a mug. 2. Pour hot water over the herbs. 3. Cover and steep for 8–10 minutes. 4. Strain and sip slowly after meals

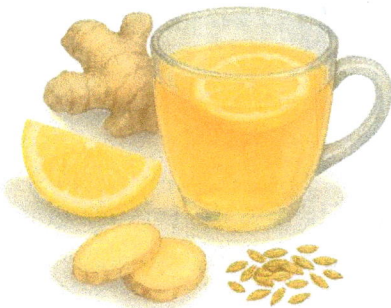

Ginger–Lemon Digestive Infusion

This warming infusion stimulates digestive fire and helps the stomach process food with ease. Ginger calms queasiness, while lemon brightens the flavor and supports natural cleansing. *Tip: Best enjoyed 20–30 minutes before or after a heavy meal.*

Ingredients	Instructions
<ul><li>1 tsp fresh grated ginger</li><li>1 slice fresh lemon</li><li>1 cup hot water</li></ul>	1. Place the ginger slices in a mug. 2. Pour hot water over them and let steep for 5 minutes. 3. Add the lemon slice, stir, and enjoy warm.

Chamomile & Anise Tea

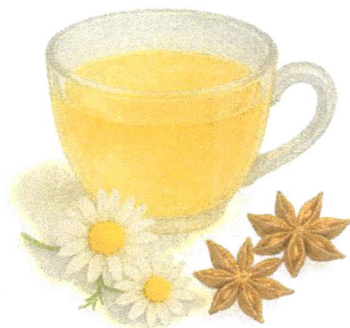

This floral-spiced blend calms stomach spasms and helps ease abdominal cramping. Chamomile soothes tension, while anise supports gentle relaxation of the digestive tract, making it ideal after rich or heavy foods.

Ingredients	Instructions
• 1 tsp dried chamomile flowers • ½ tsp crushed anise seeds • 1 cup hot water	1. Add chamomile and anise to a teapot or mug. 2. Pour hot water over the herbs. 3. Cover and steep for 7–8 minutes, then strain.

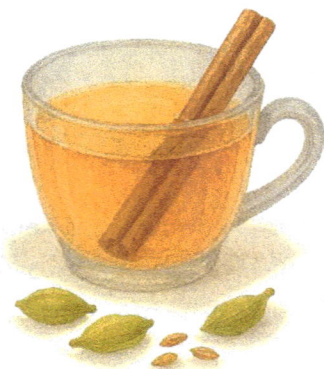

Cardamom & Cinnamon Spiced Tea

A gently spiced tea that warms the stomach and encourages natural metabolism. Cardamom aids in reducing heaviness, while cinnamon brings warmth and comfort, especially after rich meals or on cool days.

Ingredients	Instructions
• 2–3 cardamom pods (lightly crushed) • 1 small cinnamon stick • 1 cup water	1. Place cardamom pods and cinnamon stick in a small pot. 2. Add water and bring to a gentle simmer for 8–10 minutes. 3. Strain and sip warm.

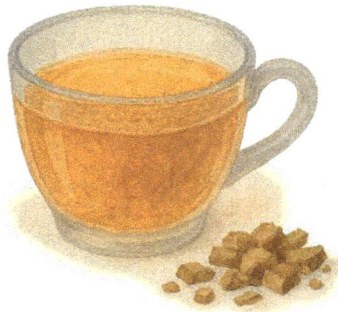

Dandelion Root Digestive Tea

This earthy tea supports both the stomach and the liver. Dandelion root gently stimulates digestion and helps the body handle heavy foods with more ease. **Safety**: *Avoid if you have gallbladder obstruction or are allergic to plants in the daisy family.*

Ingredients	Instructions
• 1 tbsp dried dandelion root (chopped) • 1 cup hot water	1. Place dandelion root in a small pot with water. 2. Bring to a gentle simmer for 10 minutes. 3. Strain and enjoy warm.

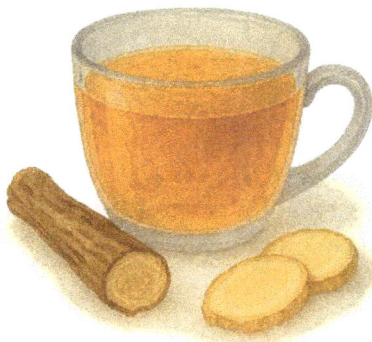

Licorice Root & Ginger Decoction

A soothing decoction that calms an irritated stomach and eases mild nausea. Licorice root coats and comforts, while ginger brings warmth and supports smoother digestion. *Safety: Avoid licorice if you have high blood pressure or heart conditions.*

Ingredients	Instructions
• 1 tsp dried licorice root pieces • 1 tsp fresh ginger slices • 1½ cups water	1. Place licorice root and ginger in a small pot with water. 2. Simmer gently for 12–15 minutes. 3. Strain into a cup and drink warm.

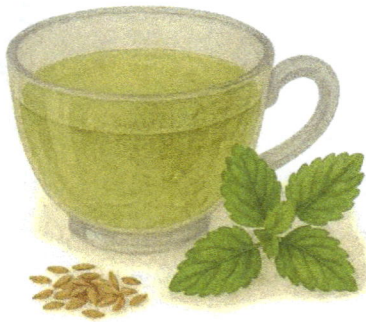

Caraway & Lemon Balm Digestive Tonic

This fragrant tonic lightens the feeling of fullness and soothes mild stomach tension. Carway seeds ease bloating, while lemon balm provides a calm, gentle balance.

Ingredients	Instructions
<ul><li>1 tsp caraway seeds (crushed)</li><li>1 tsp dried lemon balm leaves</li><li>1 cup hot water</li></ul>	1. Add caraway seeds and lemon balm to a teapot. 2. Pour hot water and cover. 3. Steep for 8–10 minutes, strain, and sip slowly.

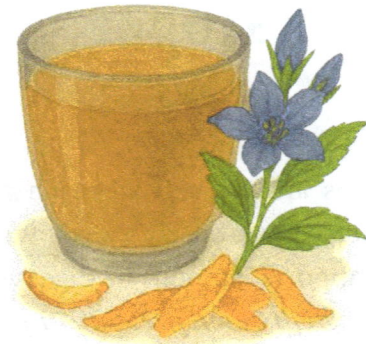

Bitters Blend with Gentian & Orange Peel

A traditional digestive tonic that stimulates natural enzyme production and prepares the stomach for meals. The bitter notes of gentian root pair with the citrus lift of orange peel, awakening digestion before eating.

Ingredients	Instructions
<ul><li>½ tsp dried gentian root</li><li>1 tsp dried orange peel</li><li>1 cup hot water</li></ul>	1. Place gentian root and orange peel in a mug. 2. Cover with hot water. 3. Steep for 5–7 minutes, then strain.

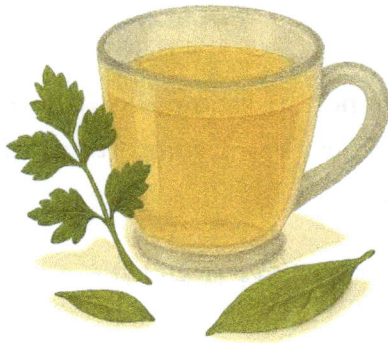

Bone Broth with Parsley & Bay Leaf

A warm, nourishing broth that comforts the stomach and supports overall digestive health. Parsley adds freshness and aids cleansing, while bay leaf brings depth and warmth.

Ingredients	Instructions
• 2–3 chicken or beef bones • 2–3 fresh parsley sprigs • 1 bay leaf • 4 cups water	1. Place bones in a large pot with water. 2. Add parsley and bay leaf. 3. Simmer gently for 2–3 hours. 4. Strain and sip warm or use as a soup base.

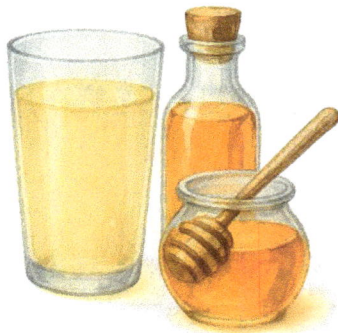

Apple Cider Vinegar & Honey Tonic

A simple tonic that helps the stomach reset and supports healthy gut balance. The mild acidity of apple cider vinegar stimulates digestion, while honey provides natural sweetness and comfort. **Tip**: *Start with a smaller amount of vinegar if you are new to its taste.*

Ingredients	Instructions
• 1 cup warm water • 1 tsp apple cider vinegar (raw, unfiltered) • 1 tsp honey	1. Add apple cider vinegar to a glass of warm water. 2. Stir in honey until dissolved. 3. Drink slowly before or after meals.

Ginger Chew for Nausea

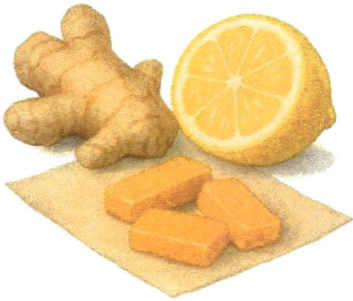

A quick, portable remedy for motion sickness or sudden nausea. Chewy ginger pieces deliver a warm, comforting taste that helps settle the stomach on the go.

Safety: *Limit intake if you have sensitive stomach lining or use blood-thinning medication.*

Ingredients	Instructions
 • ¼ cup fresh ginger juice • ½ cup honey • 1 tbsp lemon juice	1. In a small pan, warm honey and ginger juice over low heat. 2. Stir in lemon juice and simmer until thick and sticky. 3. Pour onto parchment paper, let cool, and cut into small bite-sized pieces.

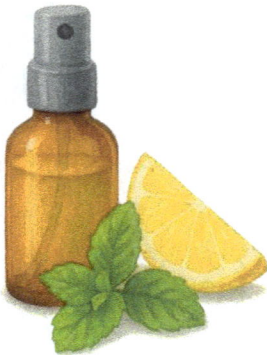

Mint & Lemon Digestive Spray

A refreshing spray that can ease mild nausea or bloating during the day. The cooling scent of peppermint combines with the brightness of lemon for quick relief you can carry in your bag.

Ingredients	Instructions
• ½ cup distilled water • 5 drops peppermint essential oil • 3 drops lemon essential oil	1. Pour water into a small spray bottle. 2. Add peppermint and lemon essential oils. 3. Shake well before each use. 4. Spray lightly in the air and breathe deeply.

Carrot & Fennel Smoothie

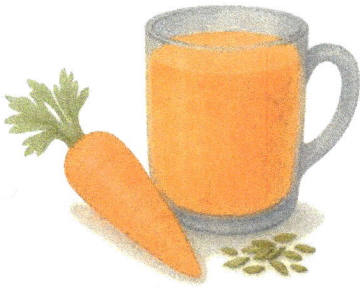

This bright orange drink is gentle on the stomach and provides natural fiber to support regular digestion. Carrots add nourishment, while fennel seeds help ease bloating and promote comfort.

Ingredients	Instructions
• 1 medium carrot (chopped) • 1 tsp fennel seeds (soaked, lightly crushed) • 1 cup water or plant milk • 1 tsp honey (optional)	1. Add carrot, soaked fennel seeds, and liquid to a blender. 2. Blend until smooth. 3. Sweeten with honey if desired and enjoy chilled.

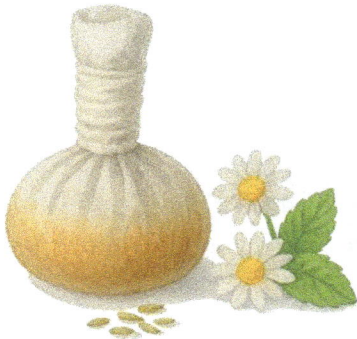

Herbal Compress for Stomach Cramps (Chamomile & Peppermint)

A simple external remedy that brings local relief during episodes of abdominal cramping. Chamomile relaxes tension, while peppermint cools and eases discomfort when applied as a warm compress. Tip: Reheat the compress by dipping it back into warm infusion as needed.

Ingredients	Instructions
• 2 tbsp dried chamomile flowers • 2 tbsp dried peppermint leaves • 2 cups hot water • 1 clean cotton cloth	1. Place chamomile and peppermint in a bowl. 2. Pour hot water over them and steep for 10 minutes. 3. Soak the cloth in the infusion, wring gently, and apply warm to the abdomen for 10–15 minutes.

Liver Detox & Metabolic Support

Your liver is one of the hardest working organs in your body. Every day it filters the blood, processes nutrients, and clears away substances you do not need. When it becomes overloaded with heavy meals, stress, or environmental toxins, you might notice signs like sluggishness, skin issues, or a general feeling of heaviness. Supporting your liver does not require drastic cleanses or expensive programs. Simple, natural remedies can provide steady support and help your body do what it already knows how to do.

This chapter focuses on practical ways to care for your liver and metabolism using accessible herbs, spices, and kitchen ingredients. The recipes are divided into clear sections so you can choose what fits best in your daily life:

- **Cleansing teas and infusions**: Gentle blends with herbs such as dandelion root, milk thistle, or nettle that encourage the liver to function smoothly and support a feeling of lightness.

- **Decoctions and tonics for metabolism**: Warm, concentrated preparations that stimulate digestion, support circulation, and help your body process energy more efficiently.

- **Smoothies and external remedies**: Nourishing drinks packed with fresh vegetables, fruits, and greens, along with soothing baths that offer an external way to release tension and encourage balance.

Most of these remedies can be made in minutes. A handful of dried herbs simmered in water becomes a simple tea that gently supports cleansing. A shot of lemon and apple cider vinegar can refresh you first thing in the morning. A beet and carrot blend offers a natural source of antioxidants that energize without relying on stimulants. Even a herbal bath can be part of metabolic care, giving your body space to relax and recover.

The idea is not to push your body into extremes but to provide it with the right support. By choosing remedies that fit into your routine, you can keep your system resilient, your digestion more efficient, and your energy balanced.

In the following pages, you will find a collection of straightforward recipes that make liver and metabolic support both practical and enjoyable. With just a few ingredients and simple steps, you can give your body the daily care it needs to stay clear, balanced, and energized.

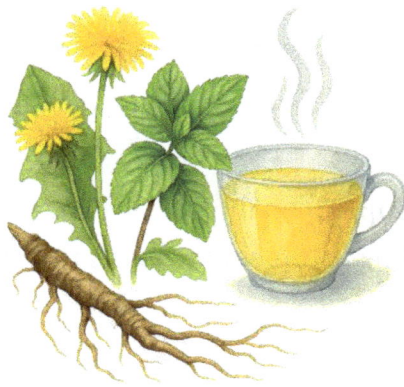

Dandelion Root & Mint Detox Tea

A light herbal tea that supports healthy liver function and brings a sense of inner freshness. Enjoy it after a heavy meal to ease digestion and promote lightness. *Safety: Avoid if you have gallbladder obstruction or allergies to plants in the daisy family.*

Ingredients	Instructions
• 1 tbsp dried dandelion root (chopped) • 1 tsp dried peppermint leaves • 1 cup hot water	1. Place the dandelion root in a small pot with the water. 2. Simmer gently for 10 minutes. 3. Remove from heat, add peppermint, and cover for 5 minutes. 4. Strain and sip warm.

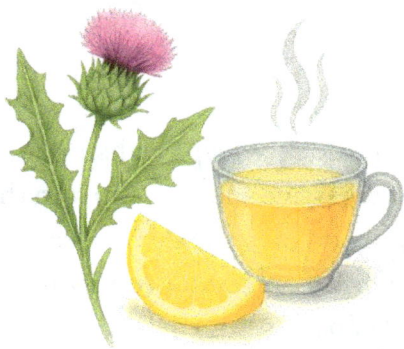

Milk Thistle & Lemon Infusion

This gentle infusion nourishes the liver and supports its natural cleansing processes. The citrus touch of lemon makes it refreshing and easy to enjoy daily. Safety: Avoid milk thistle if you are allergic to plants in the ragweed family.

Ingredients	Instructions
• 1 tsp crushed milk thistle seeds • 1 slice fresh lemon • 1 cup hot water	1. Lightly crush the milk thistle seeds. 2. Place them in a teapot and pour hot water over. 3. Add the lemon slice. 4. Cover and steep for 10 minutes, then strain.

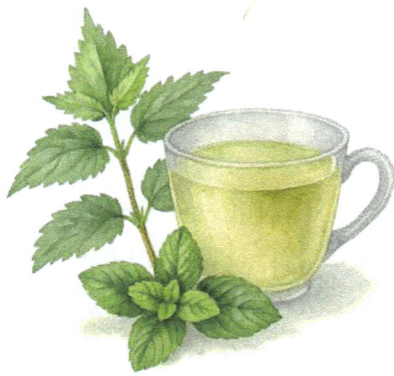

Nettle & Peppermint Liver Tea

Nettle provides minerals that support vitality and liver health, while peppermint adds a cooling lift. A simple tea to refresh the body in the afternoon.

Ingredients	Instructions
• 1 tbsp dried nettle leaves • 1 tsp dried peppermint leaves • 1 cup hot water	1. Place nettle and peppermint in a mug. 2. Pour hot water over them. 3. Cover and steep for 7–8 minutes. 4. Strain and enjoy warm or cooled.

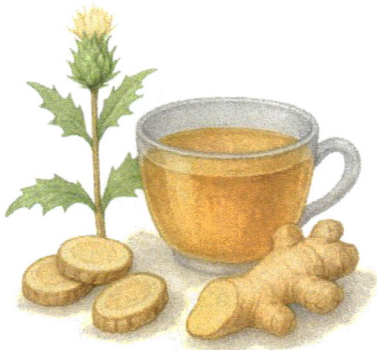

Burdock Root & Ginger Detox Brew

This warming brew combines burdock's deep cleansing properties with ginger's gentle digestive support. Sip it in the morning to stimulate circulation and help the body release toxins. *Safety: Avoid burdock during pregnancy or if you have allergies to daisies or related plants.*

Ingredients	Instructions
• 1 tbsp dried burdock root • 1 tsp fresh ginger slices • 2 cups water	1. Place burdock root and ginger in a pot with water. 2. Bring to a gentle simmer for 15–20 minutes. 3. Strain and drink warm.

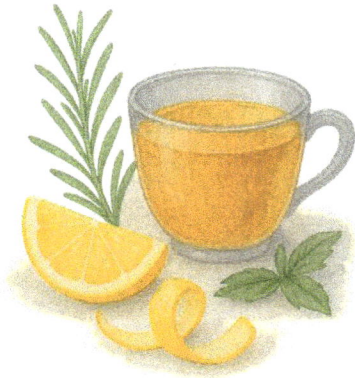

Lemon Peel & Rosemary Cleansing Tea

A refreshing blend that supports liver cleansing while awakening the senses. Lemon peel offers light detox support, and rosemary brings clarity and circulation.

Ingredients	Instructions
• 1 tsp dried lemon peel • 1 tsp dried rosemary • 1 cup hot water	1. Place lemon peel and rosemary in a cup. 2. Pour hot water over the herbs. 3. Cover and steep for 8 minutes. 4. Strain and enjoy warm.

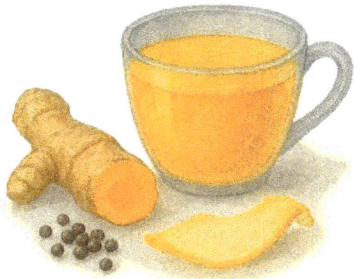

Turmeric–Black Pepper Detox Decoction

Turmeric supports natural detox and healthy metabolism, while black pepper enhances its absorption. A grounding drink to warm the body and aid digestion. *Tip: Adding a small spoon of honey can balance turmeric's earthy flavor.*

Ingredients	Instructions
• 1 tsp turmeric powder (or fresh grated turmeric) • 1 pinch black pepper • 1½ cups water	1. Add turmeric and black pepper to a pot with water. 2. Simmer gently for 10 minutes. 3. Strain and drink warm.

Cinnamon & Clove Metabolism Tonic

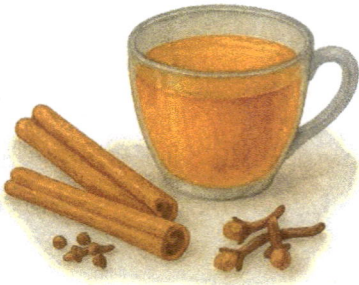

This aromatic tonic gently stimulates circulation and digestive fire. Cinnamon adds warmth, while cloves bring a spicy boost that helps energize the body. *Safety: Avoid excess clove use if you have sensitive stomach or bleeding disorders.*

Ingredients	Instructions
• 1 small cinnamon stick • 2 whole cloves • 1 cup hot water	1. Place cinnamon and cloves in a mug. 2. Pour hot water and cover. 3. Steep for 7–8 minutes. 4. Strain and sip slowly.

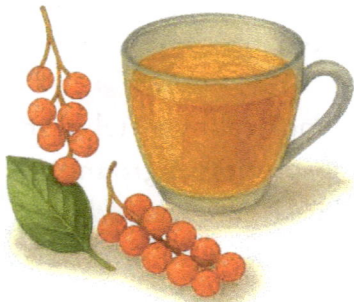

Schisandra Berry Decoction

Schisandra berries are valued for supporting liver health and resilience against stress. This tart-sweet decoction is grounding and balancing, ideal for regular use.

Safety: Avoid if pregnant or breastfeeding without medical advice.

Ingredients	Instructions
• 1 tbsp dried schisandra berries • 2 cups water	1. Place schisandra berries in a small pot with water. 2. Simmer gently for 20 minutes. 3. Strain and enjoy warm or cool.

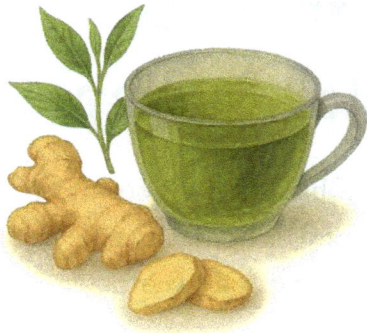

Green Tea & Ginger Metabolic Booster

A vibrant infusion that blends the clean lift of green tea with the warmth of ginger. Perfect for a natural energy boost during mid-morning or early afternoon. *Safety: Limit intake if sensitive to caffeine or using blood-thinning medication.*

Ingredients	Instructions
• 1 tsp green tea leaves • 1 tsp fresh ginger slices • 1 cup hot water	1. Place green tea leaves and ginger in a mug. 2. Pour hot water and steep for 5 minutes. 3. Strain and sip warm.

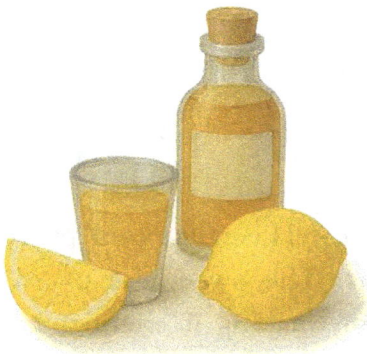

Lemon–Apple Cider Vinegar Morning Shot

A sharp, revitalizing shot that wakes digestion and supports natural cleansing. Lemon brightens the flavor while raw apple cider vinegar stimulates metabolism. *Tip: Start with a smaller amount of vinegar if you're not used to its taste.*

Ingredients	Instructions
• ½ cup warm water • 1 tsp raw apple cider vinegar • 1 tsp fresh lemon juice • 1 tsp honey (optional)	1. Add apple cider vinegar and lemon juice to the warm water. 2. Stir well. 3. Sweeten with honey if desired. 4. Drink in the morning before breakfast.

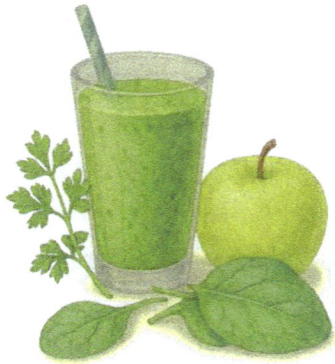

Green Detox Smoothie (Spinach, Parsley & Apple)

Packed with chlorophyll and fiber, this smoothie gently supports detox and boosts energy. Spinach and parsley nourish the body, while apple adds natural sweetness.

Ingredients	Instructions
• 1 cup fresh spinach leaves • ½ cup fresh parsley • 1 medium apple (chopped) • 1 cup water or plant milk • 1 tsp honey (optional)	1. Place spinach, parsley, apple, and liquid in a blender. 2. Blend until smooth. 3. Sweeten with honey if desired and serve fresh.

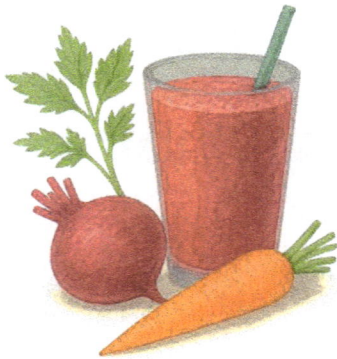

Beet & Carrot Liver Cleanser

A vibrant blend that supports natural liver detox and provides a rich source of antioxidants. The sweetness of carrot balances the earthy beet flavor, making it energizing and grounding.

Ingredients	Instructions
• 1 medium beet (peeled and chopped) • 1 medium carrot (chopped) • 1 cup water or plant milk	1. Add beet, carrot, and liquid to a blender. 2. Blend until smooth. 3. Serve immediately, chilled or at room temperature.

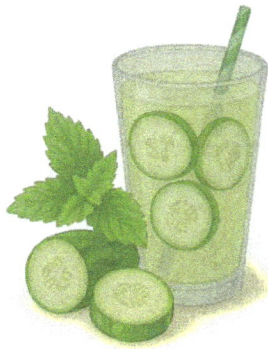

Cucumber & Mint Cooling Drink

This hydrating blend soothes the body and refreshes the liver. Cucumber cools from within, while mint supports lightness after heavy or salty meals.

Ingredients	Instructions
<ul><li>½ cucumber (sliced)</li><li>1 tbsp fresh mint leaves</li><li>1 cup cold water</li></ul>	1. Place cucumber slices and mint in a glass or jar. 2. Pour cold water over them. 3. Let infuse for 10 minutes before drinking.

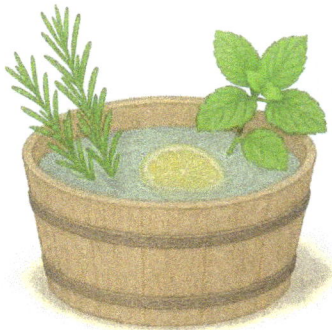

Herbal Detox Bath

This soothing bath blend helps the body release tension while supporting gentle detox. Rosemary stimulates circulation, and lemon balm calms the nervous system, leaving you refreshed.

Ingredients	Instructions
<ul><li>½ cup dried rosemary</li><li>½ cup dried lemon balm leaves</li><li>1 muslin bag or clean cotton cloth</li><li>Warm bathwater</li></ul>	1. Place rosemary and lemon balm in the muslin bag. 2. Tie securely and drop into warm bathwater. 3. Let steep for 5 minutes, then soak for 20 minutes.

Blood Sugar & Cravings Balance

Maintaining balanced blood sugar is one of the simplest ways to feel steady, focused, and in control of your energy. When your levels swing too quickly, you may notice sudden crashes, irritability, or strong cravings for sweets. These ups and downs can make it difficult to stay productive, leaving you tired in the afternoon and restless at night. While processed snacks or sugary drinks might seem like an easy fix, they often make the cycle worse.

This chapter is designed to give you natural, practical remedies that help stabilize blood sugar and manage cravings in everyday life. The recipes are organized into three clear sections that cover the most common needs:

- **Balancing teas and infusions**: Gentle blends with herbs and spices such as cinnamon, fenugreek, or bilberry leaves that support stable energy and ease digestive strain after meals.

- **Functional tonics and decoctions**: Concentrated preparations with ingredients like bitter melon, licorice root, or mulberry that are traditionally used to encourage healthy glucose processing and metabolic support.

- **Everyday craving remedies**: Smoothies, snacks, and simple drinks that keep you satisfied, calm sugar spikes, and provide natural alternatives to processed sweets.

The strength of these remedies is their simplicity. You do not need complicated tools or rare ingredients. A teaspoon of seeds, a stick of cinnamon, or a piece of fresh ginger can be enough to create a drink that steadies your energy and helps you avoid reaching for unhealthy snacks.

These recipes are also flexible. Some are quick options to prepare in a mug or glass when you need immediate support. Others, like nourishing smoothies or small energy bites, can be made ahead of time and kept ready for busy days.

The goal is not to avoid sugar completely but to support your body in managing it more effectively. When your blood sugar is stable, you feel calmer, less reactive, and more in control of your choices.

In the following pages, you will find clear, accessible recipes that can become part of your daily rhythm. Each one is designed to be easy, practical, and supportive, helping you create steadier energy and fewer cravings throughout the day.

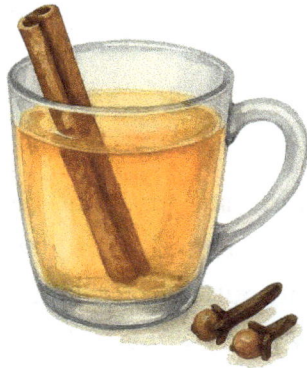

Cinnamon & Clove Balancing Tea

A warming tea that helps steady blood sugar after meals. Cinnamon enhances insulin sensitivity, while cloves add a grounding spice that curbs sweet cravings. *Tip: Enjoy after lunch or dinner to support balanced energy.*

Ingredients	Instructions
• 1 small Ceylon cinnamon stick • 2 whole cloves • 1 cup hot water	1. Place the cinnamon stick and cloves in a mug. 2. Pour hot water over them. 3. Cover and steep for 8–10 minutes. 4. Strain and sip slowly after a meal.

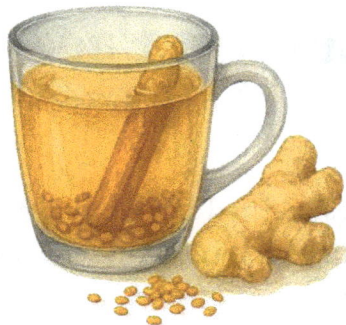

Fenugreek Seed & Ginger Infusion

This earthy infusion supports digestion and helps regulate natural blood sugar swings. Fenugreek seeds slow carbohydrate absorption, while ginger adds warmth and comfort. Safety: *Avoid fenugreek during pregnancy or if you are on blood-sugar-lowering medication without medical advice.*

Ingredients	Instructions
• 1 tsp fenugreek seeds (lightly crushed) • 1 tsp fresh ginger slices • 1 cup hot water	1. Place crushed fenugreek seeds and ginger in a teapot. 2. Pour hot water over them. 3. Cover and steep for 10 minutes. 4. Strain and drink warm.

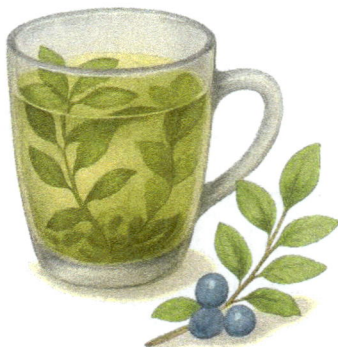

Bilberry Leaf & Green Tea Blend

Bilberry leaves provide antioxidant support that benefits circulation and blood sugar balance. Paired with green tea, this blend offers steady energy without sharp spikes. *Safety: Limit green tea if you are sensitive to caffeine.*

Ingredients	Instructions
<ul><li>1 tsp dried bilberry leaves</li><li>1 tsp green tea leaves</li><li>1 cup hot water</li></ul>	1. Place bilberry leaves and green tea in a cup. 2. Pour hot water and cover. 3. Steep for 5–7 minutes. 4. Strain and enjoy warm or cool.

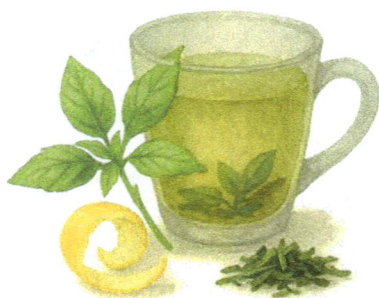

Holy Basil & Lemon Peel Tea

Holy basil (tulsi) helps calm stress-related sugar cravings, while lemon peel adds a refreshing brightness that supports digestion and metabolic balance.

Ingredients	Instructions
<ul><li>1 tbsp dried holy basil leaves</li><li>1 tsp dried lemon peel</li><li>1 cup hot water</li></ul>	1. Place holy basil and lemon peel in a mug. 2. Pour hot water over the herbs. 3. Cover and steep for 7–8 minutes. 4. Strain and sip slowly.

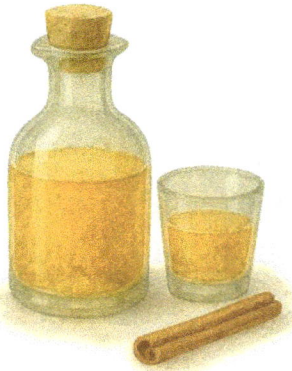

Apple Cider Vinegar & Cinnamon Morning Shot

This sharp morning shot wakes up digestion and helps balance blood sugar from the start of the day. Apple cider vinegar stimulates metabolism, while Ceylon cinnamon adds warmth and stability. *Tip: Begin with a small amount of vinegar if you're new to the taste.*

Ingredients	Instructions
• ½ cup warm water • 1 tsp raw apple cider vinegar • 1 small cinnamon stick or ½ tsp Ceylon cinnamon powder • 1 tsp honey (optional)	1. Warm the water gently. 2. Add apple cider vinegar and cinnamon. 3. Stir well, add honey if desired. 4. Drink before breakfast.

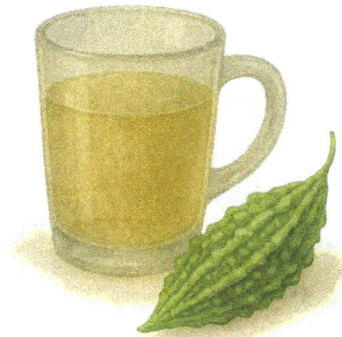

Bitter Melon Decoction

Traditionally used to support healthy blood sugar levels, bitter melon helps the body process glucose more efficiently. Its earthy, bitter flavor is balanced by slow simmering. *Safety: Avoid during pregnancy and consult your doctor if using diabetes medication.*

Ingredients	Instructions
• ½ fresh bitter melon (sliced, seeds removed) • 2 cups water	1. Place sliced bitter melon in a small pot with water. 2. Simmer gently for 10–15 minutes. 3. Strain and drink warm.

Ginger–Ceylon Cinnamon Tonic

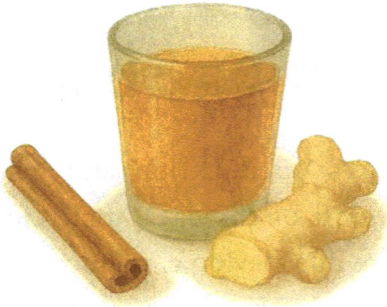

This spiced tonic stimulates metabolism and provides steady warmth without causing blood sugar spikes. A helpful drink during cool mornings or when you need gentle energy.

Ingredients	Instructions
• 1 tsp fresh ginger slices • 1 small Ceylon cinnamon stick • 1 cup water	1. Place ginger and cinnamon in a small pot with water. 2. Simmer for 8–10 minutes. 3. Strain and sip slowly.

Fenugreek & Fennel Seed Digestive Tonic

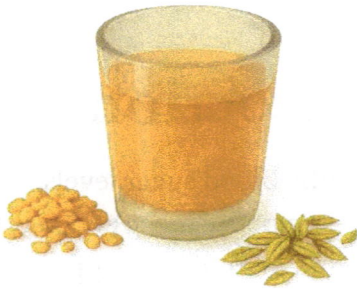

A light yet effective tonic for satiety and smoother digestion. Fenugreek supports balanced blood sugar, while fennel seeds help reduce bloating after meals. **Safety**: *Avoid fenugreek during pregnancy or with blood-sugar medication unless advised by a doctor.*

Ingredients	Instructions
• 1 tsp fenugreek seeds (soaked or lightly crushed) • 1 tsp fennel seeds • 1½ cups hot water	1. Place both types of seeds in a teapot. 2. Pour hot water and cover. 3. Steep for 10 minutes. 4. Strain and drink warm.

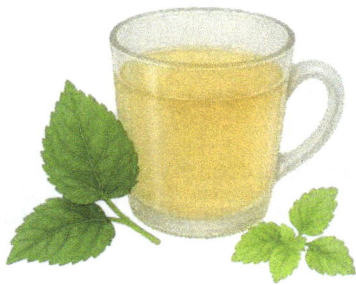

Mulberry Leaf & Lemon Balm Decoction

Mulberry leaves are known for their natural support in maintaining healthy blood sugar, while lemon balm soothes the nervous system and calms cravings.

Ingredients	Instructions
• 1 tbsp dried mulberry leaves • 1 tsp dried lemon balm leaves • 2 cups water	1. Place mulberry leaves and lemon balm in a pot with water. 2. Simmer gently for 15 minutes. 3. Strain and sip warm.

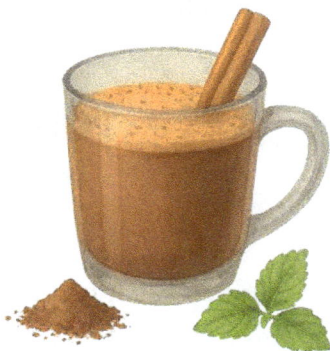

Cacao & Cinnamon Craving-Calm Drink

This rich drink satisfies sweet cravings naturally. Cacao provides magnesium and mood-supporting compounds, while Ceylon cinnamon helps steady blood sugar. *Tip: Choose raw cacao for higher antioxidant content.*

Ingredients	Instructions
• 1 cup warm milk or plant-based milk • 1 tsp raw cacao powder • ½ tsp Ceylon cinnamon powder • 1 tsp honey (optional)	1. Warm the milk gently in a pot. 2. Whisk in cacao and cinnamon. 3. Sweeten with honey if desired. 4. Drink warm as an afternoon treat.

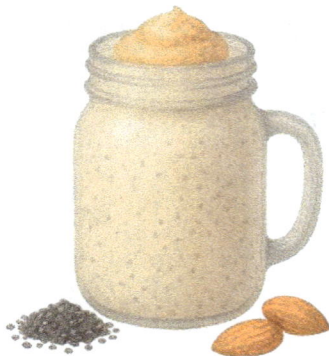

Chia Seed & Almond Milk Smoothie

Chia seeds expand in liquid to create a creamy, filling drink that helps keep blood sugar stable. Almond milk adds protein and healthy fats for steady energy.

Ingredients	Instructions
<ul><li>2 tbsp chia seeds</li><li>1 cup almond milk (unsweetened)</li><li>1 tsp honey or maple syrup (optional)</li><li>A pinch of ground cinnamon</li></ul>	1. Add chia seeds to the almond milk. 2. Stir well and let rest for 10–15 minutes to thicken. 3. Add honey or maple syrup and cinnamon if desired. 4. Stir again before drinking.

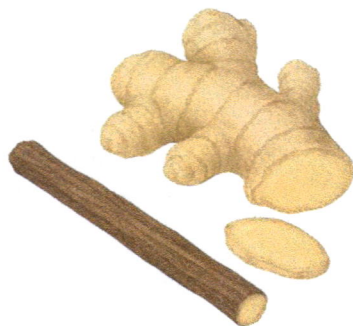

Licorice & Ginger Herbal Chew

A naturally sweet chew that can ease sudden sugar cravings and soothe the stomach. Licorice brings a pleasant flavor and supports balance, while ginger adds warmth.

Ingredients	Instructions
<ul><li>¼ cup dried licorice root (ground or powdered)</li><li>1 tbsp fresh ginger juice</li><li>¼ cup honey</li></ul>	1. In a small pan, warm honey gently. 2. Stir in ginger juice and licorice powder. 3. Simmer until thick and sticky. 4. Pour onto parchment, let cool, then cut into small chews.

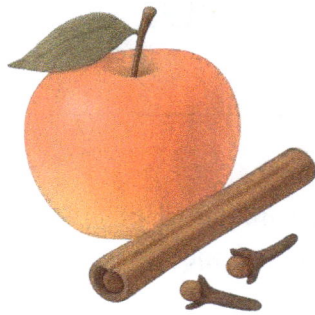

Spiced Apple Snack Infusion (Apple, Cinnamon & Clove)

This cozy infusion tastes like warm apple cider and helps ease sugar cravings. Apple adds natural sweetness, while cinnamon and cloves bring grounding warmth.

Ingredients	Instructions
• ½ apple (sliced) • 1 small Ceylon cinnamon stick • 2 whole cloves • 1 cup hot water	1. Place apple slices, cinnamon, and cloves in a teapot. 2. Pour hot water over them. 3. Cover and steep for 10 minutes. 4. Strain and enjoy warm.

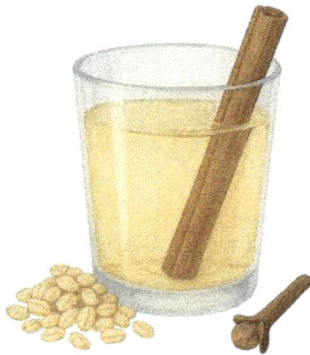

Barley & Cinnamon Cooling Infusion

A light and refreshing drink that helps regulate blood sugar while keeping you hydrated. Barley water supports steady energy release, while Ceylon cinnamon adds warmth and balance, making it a simple option for mid-day cravings.

Ingredients	Instructions
• 2 tbsp pearl barley • 1 small Ceylon cinnamon stick • 2 cups water • 1 tsp honey or lemon juice (optional)	1. Rinse the barley under running water. 2. Place barley and cinnamon stick in a small pot with water. 3. Bring to a gentle boil, then simmer for 15–20 minutes. 4. Strain into a glass or mug. 5. Add honey or lemon juice if desired, and drink warm or cooled.

Thyroid & Adrenal Support

Energy is not just about how much you sleep or how much coffee you drink. Much of your vitality is guided by two small but powerful systems inside your body: the thyroid and the adrenal glands. They influence metabolism, hormone balance, and the way you respond to stress. When they are under pressure, you may notice changes such as feeling unusually tired, struggling to focus, or finding it difficult to manage everyday challenges.

Daily life puts these systems to the test. Rushing through meals, working late into the night, or living in a constant state of alert can leave your body with fewer resources to keep its balance. Over time, this can show up as fatigue that does not improve with rest, irritability, or difficulty handling stress. While medical guidance is always important if you suspect thyroid or adrenal conditions, there are also gentle, natural ways to support these organs day by day.

In this chapter, you will explore practical remedies that provide nourishment and balance. Some are warm teas made with adaptogenic herbs such as ashwagandha, tulsi, or rhodiola, which have long been used to encourage resilience. Others are mineral-rich broths that replenish essential nutrients, or smoothies and energy bites that deliver steady fuel without overstimulating your system. You will also find simple external remedies, like aromatic steams, that refresh the mind when fatigue feels overwhelming.

The recipes are designed to be realistic and easy to prepare. Most require no more than a small pot, a jar, or a blender. You can steep a spoonful of dried leaves in hot water, blend a few nourishing ingredients into a smoothie, or prepare a tonic to sip slowly during the day. The goal is to give your body gentle, consistent support so it can maintain its natural rhythm.

As you turn the pages, you will discover preparations that fit smoothly into everyday life. Choose the ones that match your needs, whether it is a morning drink to start the day with stable energy, a midday infusion to restore calm, or an evening blend that helps you release tension. These remedies are not about quick fixes but about building small habits that keep your energy balanced and your system supported over time.

Ashwagandha & Cinnamon Balancing Tea

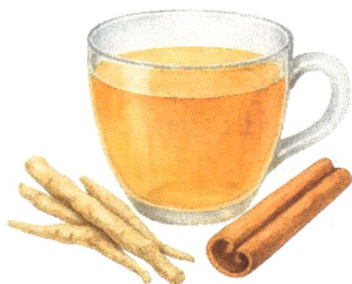

A warming tea that helps sustain energy and ease feelings of chronic fatigue. Ashwagandha supports adrenal balance, while cinnamon adds a comforting spice that steadies energy levels. Enjoy it mid-afternoon to prevent energy crashes. Safety: Avoid ashwagandha if pregnant, breastfeeding, or taking thyroid medication without medical advice.

Ingredients	Instructions
• 1 tsp dried ashwagandha root (cut or powdered) • 1 small Ceylon cinnamon stick or ½ tsp ground cinnamon • 1 cup hot water	1. Place ashwagandha and cinnamon in a mug or teapot. 2. Pour hot water over the herbs. 3. Cover and steep for 10 minutes. 4. Strain and sip warm.

Licorice Root & Ginger Infusion

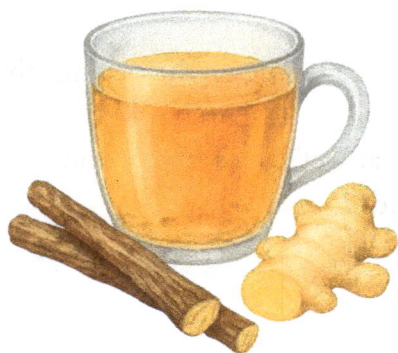

This gently spiced infusion supports vitality and helps sustain energy through the day. Licorice root soothes and nourishes the adrenal glands, while ginger provides a natural warming lift. *Safety: Avoid licorice if you have high blood pressure, kidney issues, or are pregnant.*

Ingredients	Instructions
• 1 tsp dried licorice root (chopped) • 1 tsp fresh ginger slices • 1 cup hot water	1. Place licorice root and ginger in a mug. 2. Pour hot water over them. 3. Cover and steep for 8–10 minutes. 4. Strain and enjoy warm.

Nettle & Lemon Balm Support Tea

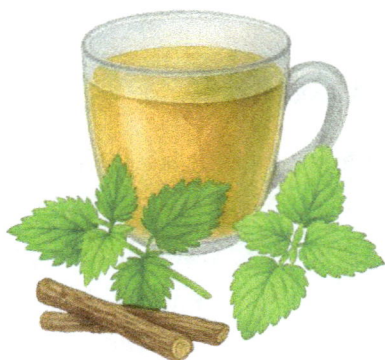

Nettle brings a rich supply of minerals that help combat fatigue, while lemon balm adds a calming touch that eases stress. This blend is a gentle way to support thyroid and adrenal balance throughout the day.

Ingredients	Instructions
• 1 tbsp dried nettle leaves • 1 tsp dried lemon balm leaves • 1 cup hot water	1. Add nettle and lemon balm to a teapot. 2. Pour hot water and cover. 3. Steep for 8–10 minutes. 4. Strain and sip slowly.

Tulsi & Mint Refreshing Infusion

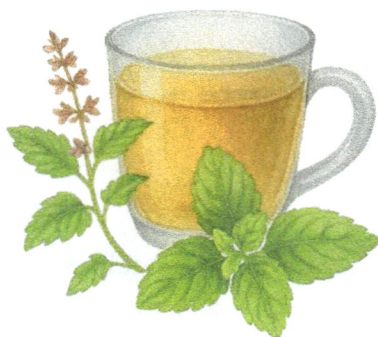

Tulsi, or holy basil, is a gentle adaptogen that calms the nervous system and supports resilience. Paired with mint, it creates a cooling infusion that refreshes the mind and promotes clarity. Perfect for mid-day balance.

Ingredients	Instructions
• 1 tbsp dried tulsi leaves • 1 tsp fresh mint leaves • 1 cup hot water	1. Place tulsi and mint in a mug. 2. Pour hot water over them. 3. Cover and steep for 7 minutes. 4. Strain and drink warm or cool.

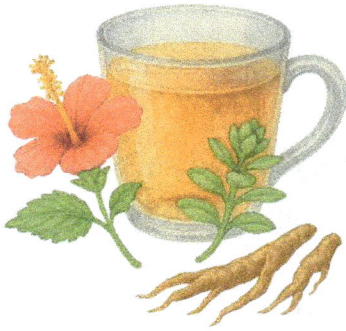

Rhodiola & Hibiscus Decoction

Rhodiola supports stress resilience and endurance, while hibiscus adds a tart, refreshing flavor rich in antioxidants. This decoction is ideal for long days when you need sustained energy. **Safety:** *Avoid rhodiola in case of uncontrolled high blood pressure or during pregnancy unless advised by a doctor.*

Ingredients	Instructions
• 1 tbsp dried rhodiola root slices • 1 tbsp dried hibiscus petals • 2 cups water	1. Place rhodiola root in a small pot with water. 2. Simmer gently for 15 minutes. 3. Remove from heat, add hibiscus, and steep 5 minutes. 4. Strain and sip warm or cooled.

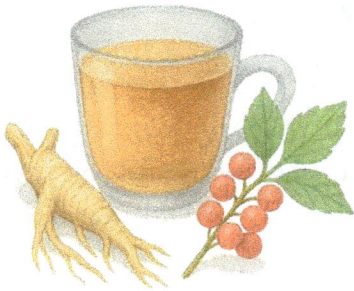

Ginseng & Schisandra Vitality Tonic

This energizing tonic combines ginseng's ability to enhance stamina with schisandra's adaptogenic support. It helps sharpen concentration while nourish

Ingredients	Instructions
• 1 tsp dried ginseng root slices • 1 tbsp dried schisandra berries • 2 cups water • 1 tsp honey (optional)	1. Place ginseng and schisandra in a pot with water. 2. Simmer gently for 20 minutes. 3. Strain and pour into a mug. 4. Add honey if desired and sip slowly.

Seaweed & Ginger Mineral Broth

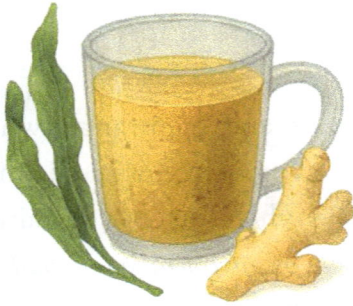

This mineral-rich broth combines the nourishing properties of seaweed with the warming support of ginger. It's a comforting way to replenish energy and provide nutrients that benefit thyroid function. **Safety:** *Avoid excess seaweed if you have thyroid disorders without medical supervision.*

Ingredients	Instructions
• 1 strip dried kelp or wakame • 2 cups water • 3–4 slices fresh ginger	1. Place kelp and ginger in a pot with water. 2. Bring to a gentle simmer for 15 minutes. 3. Remove the kelp, strain the broth, and sip warm.

Maca & Cacao Adaptogenic Drink

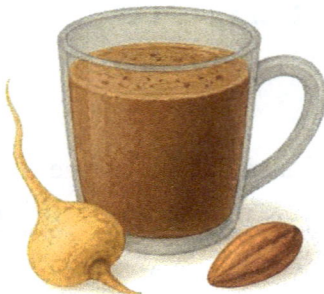

This creamy drink blends maca's grounding energy with cacao's uplifting richness. It supports hormonal balance and enhances mental focus, making it a perfect afternoon or pre-workout boost. **Tip**: *Choose raw cacao for higher antioxidant content.*

Ingredients	Instructions
• 1 cup warm milk or plant-based milk • 1 tsp maca powder • 1 tsp raw cacao powder • 1 tsp honey or maple syrup (optional)	1. Warm the milk gently in a pot. 2. Stir in maca and cacao until smooth. 3. Add honey or maple syrup if desired. 4. Drink slowly and enjoy.

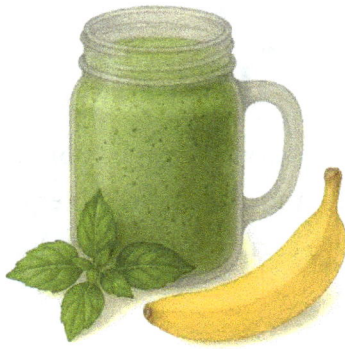

Holy Basil Morning Smoothie

A light, nourishing smoothie that supports calm energy without overstimulation. Tulsi balances the adrenal response, while fresh fruit and greens provide a steady release of nutrients. **Safety**: *Avoid tulsi during pregnancy unless guided by a healthcare professional.*

Ingredients	Instructions
• 1 cup unsweetened almond milk • 1 banana • 1 tbsp dried or fresh tulsi leaves (lightly steeped in hot water, cooled) • ½ cup fresh spinach • 1 tsp honey (optional)	1. Brew tulsi leaves in ½ cup hot water for 5 minutes, then cool. 2. Combine cooled tulsi infusion, almond milk, banana, and spinach in a blender. 3. Blend until smooth. 4. Sweeten with honey if desired and serve fresh.

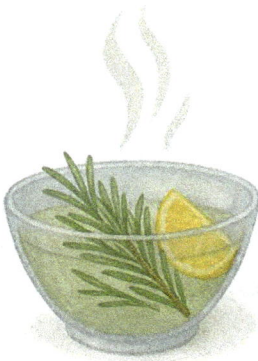

Rosemary & Lemon Vitality Steam

This fragrant steam awakens the senses and offers gentle stimulation for times of fatigue. Rosemary clears the mind, while lemon refreshes and lifts mood, making it a quick reset for tired afternoons. **Tip**: *Keep eyes closed during inhalation to avoid irritation.*

Ingredients	Instructions
• 2 tsp dried rosemary • Zest of ½ fresh lemon • 3 cups hot water • Towel	1. Place rosemary and lemon zest in a large bowl. 2. Pour hot water over them. 3. Lean over carefully with a towel over your head. 4. Inhale the steam deeply for 5–10 minutes.

Adaptogenic Energy Bites (Dates, Maca & Nuts)

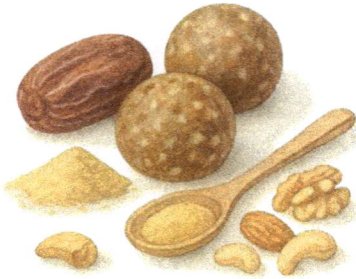

These chewy bites combine the natural sweetness of dates with maca's balancing properties and the steady energy of nuts. They're a convenient snack to carry for mid-day slumps or busy mornings.

Ingredients	Instructions
• 1 cup pitted dates • 2 tbsp maca powder • ½ cup mixed nuts (almonds, walnuts, or cashews)	1. Place dates and nuts in a food processor. 2. Blend until sticky and crumbly. 3. Add maca powder and pulse again. 4. Roll the mixture into small bite-sized balls. 5. Store in an airtight container in the fridge.

Ginger–Turmeric Warming Shot

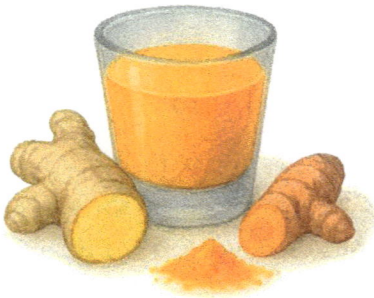

A concentrated shot that combines ginger's warmth with turmeric's balancing support. It's a quick option when you need an instant lift during stressful days. **Safety**: *Avoid high doses of turmeric if you are on blood-thinning medication.*

Ingredients	Instructions
• 1 inch fresh ginger root (grated) • ½ tsp turmeric powder • Juice of ½ lemon • ½ cup water	1. Blend ginger, turmeric, lemon juice, and water until smooth. 2. Strain if desired. 3. Drink immediately as a small shot.

Ashwagandha & Honey Night Drink

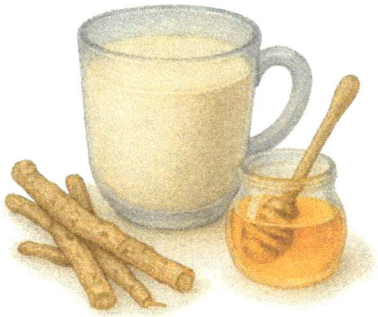

A gentle evening drink that soothes the nervous system and supports nightly recovery. Ashwagandha promotes balance, while honey adds calming sweetness, making it an ideal way to wind down before sleep. **Safety**: *Avoid ashwagandha if pregnant or on thyroid medication unless advised by a healthcare professional.*

Ingredients	Instructions
• 1 cup warm milk or plant-based milk • 1 tsp ashwagandha powder • 1 tsp raw honey	1. Warm the milk gently in a small pot. 2. Stir in ashwagandha powder until fully dissolved. 3. Remove from heat, add honey, and sip slowly.

Lemon Balm & Brazil Nut Evening Smoothie

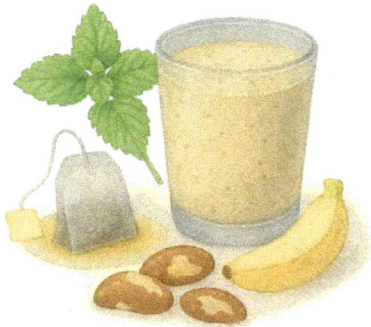

This creamy evening blend combines the gentle calm of lemon balm with the selenium-rich nourishment of Brazil nuts, which are known to support thyroid function. It's a soothing way to wind down while giving your body key minerals for hormonal balance. **Safety**: *Limit Brazil nut intake to a few pieces per day to avoid excessive selenium.*

Ingredients	Instructions
• 1 cup unsweetened oat milk • 1 tsp dried lemon balm (lightly steeped and cooled) • 2–3 Brazil nuts (soaked overnight) • ½ banana • 1 tsp honey (optional)	1. Steep lemon balm in ½ cup hot water for 7 minutes, then cool. 2. Add the cooled infusion, oat milk, soaked Brazil nuts, and banana to a blender. 3. Blend until smooth and creamy. 4. Sweeten with honey if desired. Serve slightly chilled.

Share Your Experience

This book is filled with remedies, but the real value lies in how they work for you. Each reader's path looks a little different: for one, it might be finally sleeping through the night after weeks of restlessness; for another, it could be the simple comfort of easing tension after a stressful day; for someone else, it may just be discovering a morning ritual that sets a calmer tone for the day ahead.

That variety of experiences is what brings these pages to life. And that's why your feedback matters so much. When you leave a review, you're not only sharing your personal journey, you're helping others who are standing right where you once stood, curious but uncertain about whether these remedies truly fit into everyday life.

I read every review personally, all of them, whether they are full of enthusiasm or point out what didn't work as expected. Both are equally valuable. Positive feedback shows me what resonates, while critical notes guide me to improve and make future editions even more useful.

Your review doesn't need to be long or polished. A few honest lines about which remedy you tried, how it felt, or what stood out to you is more than enough. That single comment may be the encouragement another reader needs to try their first calming tea or to believe that something so simple can make a real difference.

It takes less than a minute to write, yet the ripple effect can be profound. Your words become part of a community effort, readers helping readers, one experience at a time.

Thank you for considering it. Your voice matters, and your perspective can light the way for someone else seeking balance.

Scan to leave a review

Women's Wellness (Cycle, PMS & Menopause)

W omen's health moves in rhythms that shift over time. Each stage of life brings unique needs, and the body often signals these changes through cycles, transitions, and physical sensations. Paying attention to these signals and responding with practical support can make everyday life smoother and more balanced.

During the menstrual cycle, many women notice discomfort such as cramps, bloating, or mood changes. These moments do not always require medication. Sometimes a warm tea, a simple compress, or a refreshing herbal infusion is enough to ease tension and help you feel more comfortable. Small practices like these can turn difficult days into more manageable ones.

As energy levels fluctuate throughout the month, certain plants can provide steady nourishment. Ingredients such as maca, ashwagandha, or sesame seeds can be blended into drinks or snacks, supporting both vitality and emotional stability. These remedies are designed to be easy additions to your daily routine, offering practical ways to stay balanced even on demanding days.

Later in life, menopause brings its own set of changes. Hot flashes, sleep disturbances, and shifts in mood are common experiences during this stage. Here too, natural remedies can make a difference. Cooling teas with sage or red clover, soothing baths with rose or lavender, and nutrient-rich smoothies with flaxseeds or berries can all provide gentle, accessible support.

What unites these remedies is their simplicity. You do not need complicated techniques or rare ingredients. Most of the recipes can be prepared in minutes with herbs and foods you may already keep in your kitchen. A slice of lemon, a pinch of cinnamon, or a handful of seeds can become an effective way to care for your body.

As you explore this chapter, think of it as a toolkit that adapts to your needs at different times in life. Whether you are looking for relief during your cycle, steady energy during busy days, or comfort through menopause, the following pages will offer clear, practical recipes you can rely on.

Ginger & Cinnamon Warm Relief Tea

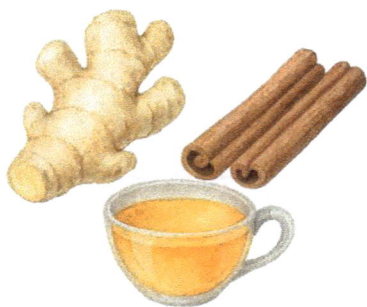

A soothing tea that combines the warming spice of ginger with the comforting sweetness of cinnamon. It helps ease menstrual cramps and brings a gentle sense of warmth to the body, making it perfect for cold days or when you need comfort during your cycle. **Tip**: *Enjoy with a warm compress on your abdomen for extra relief.*

Ingredients	Instructions
<ul><li>1 tsp fresh grated ginger</li><li>1 small Ceylon cinnamon stick or ½ tsp ground cinnamon</li><li>1 cup hot water</li><li>1 tsp honey (optional)</li></ul>	1. Place ginger and cinnamon in a mug. 2. Pour hot water over the ingredients. 3. Cover and steep for 7–8 minutes. 4. Strain and sip slowly, adding honey if desired.

Raspberry Leaf & Rose Tea

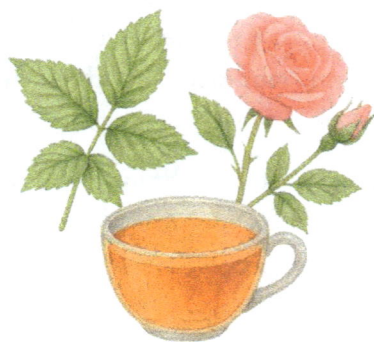

This floral tea supports uterine tone and provides a sense of balance during the menstrual cycle. Raspberry leaf gently nurtures the reproductive system, while rose petals lift the mood with their delicate fragrance. **Safety**: *Avoid raspberry leaf tea during pregnancy unless guided by a healthcare professional.*

Ingredients	Instructions
<ul><li>1 tbsp dried raspberry leaves</li><li>1 tsp dried rose petals</li><li>1 cup hot water</li></ul>	1. Place raspberry leaves and rose petals in a teapot or mug. 2. Pour hot water over them. 3. Cover and steep for 8–10 minutes. 4. Strain and enjoy warm.

Chamomile & Fennel Comfort Tea

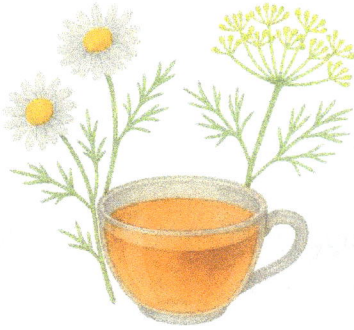

A gentle blend that soothes bloating and calms abdominal tension. Chamomile eases discomfort, while fennel supports digestion and reduces gas, making this tea ideal during PMS or menstrual days.

Ingredients	Instructions
<ul><li>1 tsp dried chamomile flowers</li><li>1 tsp fennel seeds (lightly crushed)</li><li>1 cup hot water</li></ul>	1. Add chamomile and fennel to a cup. 2. Pour hot water over the herbs. 3. Cover and steep for 7 minutes. 4. Strain and sip warm after meals or when cramps arise.

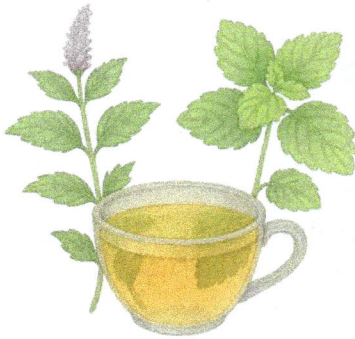

Peppermint & Lemon Balm Tummy Relief Infusion

Refreshing and calming, this infusion helps soothe digestive upset and ease tension in the stomach during the menstrual cycle. Peppermint provides a cooling effect, while lemon balm relaxes the body and mind.

Ingredients	Instructions
<ul><li>1 tsp dried peppermint leaves</li><li>1 tsp dried lemon balm leaves</li><li>1 cup hot water</li></ul>	1. Combine peppermint and lemon balm in a mug. 2. Pour hot water over them. 3. Cover and steep for 8 minutes. 4. Strain and drink slowly.

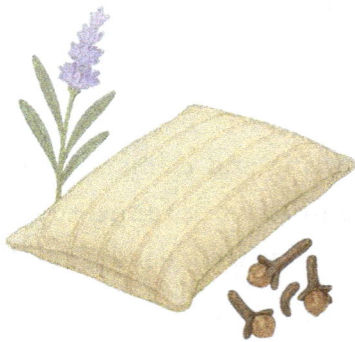

Heat Pack with Lavender & Clove

A simple external remedy to ease abdominal cramps and provide soothing warmth. Lavender calms tension, while clove offers natural warming support to relax the muscles. **Safety:** *Ensure the pouch is warm but not hot to avoid skin irritation.*

Ingredients	Instructions
<ul><li>1 small cotton or linen pouch</li><li>½ cup dried lavender flowers</li><li>1 tsp whole cloves</li><li>Clean cloth or microwave-safe heating pad</li></ul>	1. Fill the pouch with lavender and cloves. 2. Warm gently in the microwave for 20–30 seconds or place on a warm radiator. 3. Place on your lower abdomen and rest for 10–15 minutes.

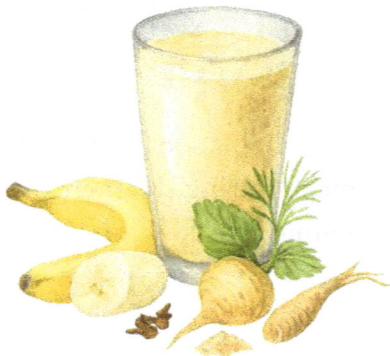

Maca & Ashwagandha Energy Smoothie

This nourishing smoothie blends maca and ashwagandha to support vitality and emotional stability. A creamy, grounding drink that helps maintain steady energy during busy or hormonally intense days. **Safety**: *Avoid ashwagandha if pregnant, breastfeeding, or taking thyroid medication without medical advice.*

Ingredients	Instructions
<ul><li>1 cup plant-based milk (almond, oat, or coconut)</li><li>1 tsp maca powder</li><li>½ tsp ashwagandha powder</li><li>1 banana</li><li>1 tsp honey or maple syrup (optional)</li></ul>	1. Place all ingredients in a blender. 2. Blend until smooth and creamy. 3. Pour into a glass and enjoy fresh.

Shatavari & Cardamom Tonic

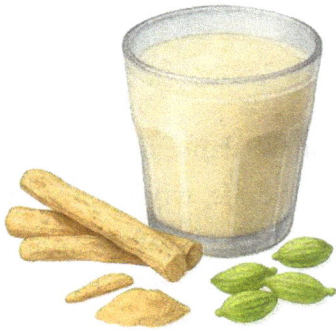

Shatavari has long been used in traditional wellness practices to support hormonal balance in women. Paired with the warm spice of cardamom, this tonic feels both nourishing and comforting. **Safety**: *Avoid shatavari during pregnancy unless guided by a healthcare professional.*

Ingredients	Instructions
• 1 tsp dried shatavari root powder	1. 1 tsp dried shatavari root powder
• 2–3 cardamom pods (lightly crushed)	2. 2–3 cardamom pods (lightly crushed)
• 1 cup warm milk or plant-based milk	3. 1 cup warm milk or plant-based milk
• 1 tsp honey (optional)	4. 1 tsp honey (optional)

Ginger–Turmeric Comfort Latte

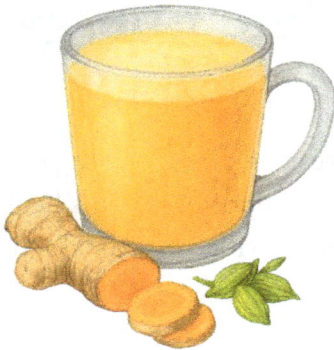

A golden latte that combines the warming spice of ginger with the soothing balance of turmeric. It supports joint comfort and eases tension during the menstrual cycle, making it an ideal evening drink. **Safety**: *Avoid high doses of turmeric if taking blood-thinning medication.*

Ingredients	Instructions
• 1 cup warm milk or plant-based milk	1. Warm the milk gently in a saucepan.
• 1 tsp grated fresh ginger	2. Stir in ginger and turmeric.
• ½ tsp turmeric powder	3. Add a pinch of black pepper to boost absorption.
• 1 pinch black pepper	4. Sweeten with honey if desired and sip warm.
• 1 tsp honey (optional)	

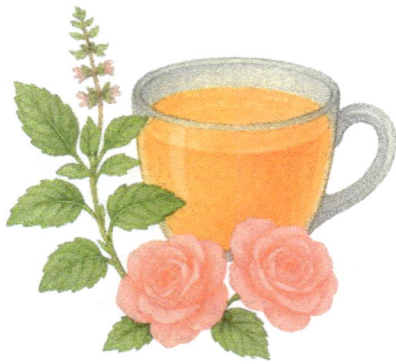

Holy Basil & Rose Balancing Tea

A fragrant tea that nurtures emotional balance and calmness. Holy basil (tulsi) supports stress resilience, while rose petals bring a soft floral note that soothes the heart. **Safety**: *Avoid holy basil during pregnancy unless advised by a healthcare professional.*

Ingredients	Instructions
<ul><li>1 tbsp dried holy basil leaves</li><li>1 tsp dried rose petals</li><li>1 cup hot water</li></ul>	1. Place holy basil and rose petals in a teapot. 2. Pour hot water over the herbs. 3. Cover and steep for 8–10 minutes. 4. Strain and drink slowly.

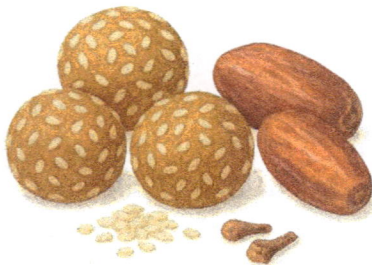

Sesame Seed & Date Energy Bits

These nourishing bites provide steady energy for long days. Sesame seeds deliver minerals that support women's health, while dates add natural sweetness and fiber for sustained vitality.

Ingredients	Instructions
<ul><li>1 cup pitted dates</li><li>½ cup sesame seeds (lightly toasted)</li><li>1 tbsp honey or nut butter (optional)</li></ul>	1. Blend dates in a food processor until sticky. 2. Add sesame seeds and honey or nut butter. 3. Mix until combined. 4. Roll into small bite-sized balls and store in an airtight container.

Sage & Lemon Balm Cooling Tea

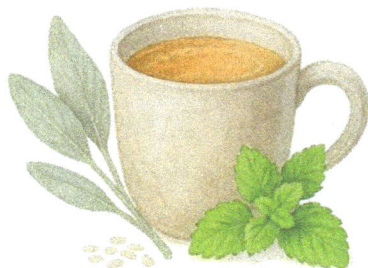

A refreshing herbal tea that helps ease hot flashes and promote calm during menopause. Sage provides cooling comfort, while lemon balm supports relaxation and emotional balance. **Safety**: *Avoid high doses of sage during pregnancy or if you have certain medical conditions such as high blood pressure or seizures.*

Ingredients	Instructions
<ul><li>1 tsp dried sage leaves</li><li>1 tsp dried lemon balm leaves</li><li>1 cup hot water</li></ul>	1. Place sage and lemon balm in a cup. 2. Pour hot water over the herbs. 3. Cover and steep for 7–8 minutes. 4. Strain and enjoy warm or cooled.

Red Clover & Mint Infusion

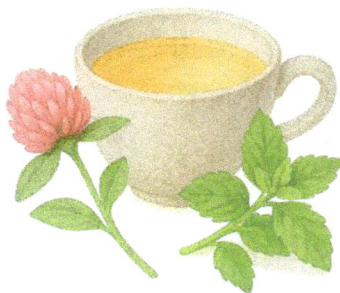

This gentle infusion supports hormonal transitions during menopause. Red clover provides phytoestrogenic support, while mint refreshes and soothes the body, easing tension and promoting comfort. **Safety**: *Avoid red clover if you have a history of estrogen-sensitive conditions or are taking blood-thinning medication.*

Ingredients	Instructions
<ul><li>1 tbsp dried red clover blossoms</li><li>1 tsp dried peppermint leaves</li><li>1 cup hot water</li></ul>	1. Place red clover and peppermint in a teapot. 2. Pour hot water over the herbs. 3. Cover and steep for 8–10 minutes. 4. Strain and sip warm or cooled.

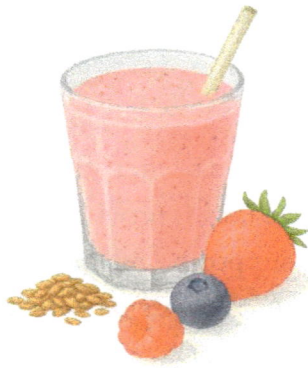

Flaxseed & Berry Smoothie

A nutrient-rich smoothie that supports hormonal health and nourishes the skin. Flaxseeds provide essential omega-3s and lignans, while berries add antioxidants and natural sweetness. **Tip**: *Use freshly ground flaxseeds to preserve nutrients.*

Rose & Lavender Relaxing

Ingredients	Instructions
• 1 cup plant-based milk or yogurt • 2 tbsp ground flaxseeds • ½ cup fresh or frozen mixed berries • 1 tsp honey or maple syrup (optional)	1. Add all ingredients to a blender. 2. Blend until smooth and creamy. 3. Pour into a glass and enjoy fresh.

Bath

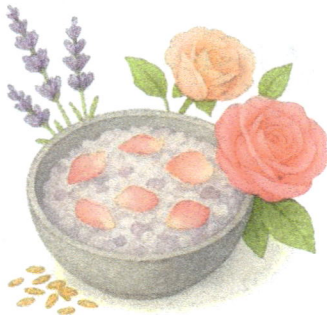

A calming bath soak that eases tension and promotes restful sleep during menopause. Rose petals soften the skin, while lavender fills the air with a soothing fragrance.

Ingredients	Instructions
• ½ cup dried rose petals • ½ cup dried lavender flowers • 1 muslin bag or clean cotton cloth • Warm bathwater	1. Place rose petals and lavender in the muslin bag. 2. Tie securely and drop into warm bathwater. 3. Let steep for 5 minutes. 4. Soak in the bath for 20 minutes, breathing deeply.

Skin, Hair & Nails Care

How your skin, hair, and nails look often reflects how your body feels inside. Dull skin, brittle nails, or tired hair can be signs of stress, poor diet, or environmental strain. While beauty products on the market promise quick fixes, many of the most effective solutions come from simple, natural ingredients that nourish, soothe, and protect from the outside in.

This chapter gathers remedies that focus on visible wellness. They are not about covering up imperfections but about supporting your body's natural ability to repair and restore. With just a few herbs, oils, and kitchen staples, you can create treatments that are gentle, affordable, and easy to prepare at home.

You will find:

- **Skin soothers** – gels, mists, and masks made with herbs such as calendula, aloe, or green tea that calm irritation and bring out natural glow.

- **Hair care blends** – rinses, masks, and serums with rosemary, nettle, hibiscus, or coconut oil to encourage strength, shine, and healthy growth.

- **Nail and hand remedies** – simple soaks, serums, and creams that support resilience, soften cuticles, and protect against dryness.

Most of these recipes can be prepared in just a few steps. A spoonful of aloe gel becomes a refreshing treatment for tired skin. A handful of rosemary steeped in water creates a mineral-rich rinse that strengthens your hair. Olive oil and lemon can be turned into a quick soak that restores brittle nails.

These are not complicated rituals that require hours of preparation. They are practical solutions that fit into your daily routine. You can apply a mask while reading, use a hand cream after washing dishes, or keep a small serum bottle by your bedside for nightly care.

By using these remedies, you are not only caring for appearance but also reinforcing the link between inner and outer balance. Healthy skin, hair, and nails can become signs that your body is being nourished and supported in simple, natural ways.

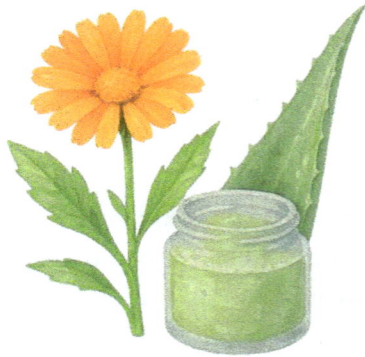

Calendula & Aloe Soothing Gel

A gentle gel that calms redness and hydrates sensitive skin. Calendula's skin-soothing qualities combine with aloe's cooling effect, making it perfect after sun exposure or to ease dryness. **Tip:** *Store up to 2 weeks in the fridge for freshness. Apply to clean skin after sun, shaving, or irritation.*

Ingredients	Instructions
• 2 tbsp aloe vera gel (fresh or store-bought, pure) • 1 tbsp calendula-infused oil • 3–4 drops lavender essential oil (optional for aroma)	1. Place aloe vera gel in a clean glass bowl. 2. Add calendula oil and whisk until smooth. 3. Stir in lavender oil if desired. 4. Transfer into a small jar and keep refrigerated.

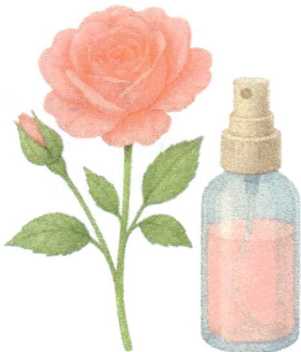

Rosewater Facial Mist

A refreshing mist that tones the skin and revives a tired complexion. The delicate fragrance of rosewater hydrates and refreshes during the day. **Tip**: *Keep in the fridge for an extra cooling effect.*

Ingredients	Instructions
• ½ cup pure rosewater • 1 tsp witch hazel (optional, for extra toning) • 1 small spray bottle	1. Pour rosewater into the spray bottle. 2. Add witch hazel if using, then shake gently. 3. Store in a cool place. Spray lightly over face when you need a boost.

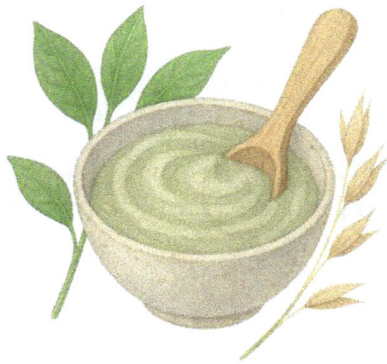

Green Tea & Oat Face Mask

This simple mask calms irritation and reduces redness. Green tea soothes the skin while oats gently soften and restore balance. **Safety**: *Always patch-test before applying to sensitive skin.*

Ingredients	Instructions
<ul><li>1 tbsp ground oats</li><li>2 tbsp cooled green tea (strong brew)</li><li>1 tsp honey</li></ul>	1. Brew a cup of strong green tea and let it cool. 2. Mix ground oats with 2 tbsp of the tea to form a paste. 3. Add honey and blend well. 4. Apply to clean face, leave for 10–15 minutes, then rinse gently.

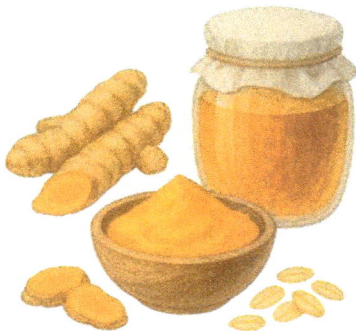

Turmeric & Honey Brightening Paste

A natural way to enhance skin glow and even tone. Turmeric adds warmth and radiance, while honey hydrates and soothes.

Ingredients	Instructions
<ul><li>1 tsp turmeric powder</li><li>1 tbsp plain yogurt (or water for sensitive skin)</li><li>1 tsp raw honey</li></ul>	1. Combine turmeric and yogurt in a small bowl. 2. Add honey and mix until smooth. 3. Apply a thin layer to clean skin. 4. Leave for 8–10 minutes, then rinse thoroughly.

Chamomile & Cucumber Under-Eye Compress

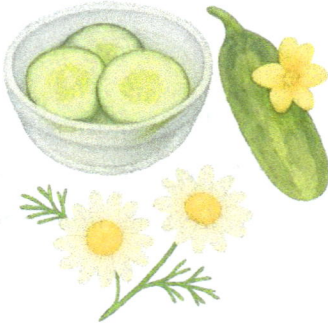

A cooling compress that reduces puffiness and soothes tired eyes. Chamomile calms the skin, while cucumber hydrates and refreshes. **Tip:** *Chill the cucumber slices for extra soothing relief.*

Ingredients	Instructions
<ul><li>2 tbsp dried chamomile flowers (or 2 tea bags)</li><li>½ cucumber, sliced</li><li>1 cup hot water</li><li>2 cotton pads or cloth squares</li></ul>	1. Brew chamomile tea with hot water; let cool slightly. 2. Soak cotton pads in the tea. 3. Place a cucumber slice on each pad. 4. Rest them over closed eyes for 10 minutes.

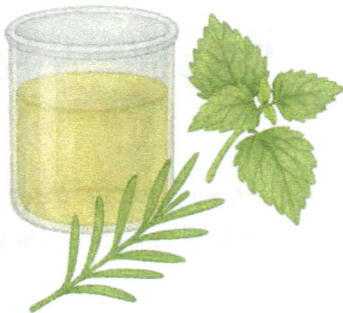

Rosemary & Nettle Hair Rinse

A herbal rinse that strengthens hair and encourages growth. Rosemary boosts circulation to the scalp, while nettle nourishes with minerals. **Tip:** *Use once or twice a week for best results.*

Ingredients	Instructions
<ul><li>1 tbsp dried rosemary</li><li>1 tbsp dried nettle leaves</li><li>2 cups hot water</li></ul>	1. Place rosemary and nettle in a heat-proof jar. 2. Pour hot water over the herbs and cover. 3. Steep for 15–20 minutes, then strain. 4. After shampooing, pour the cooled rinse through your hair.

Coconut Oil & Hibiscus Hair Mask

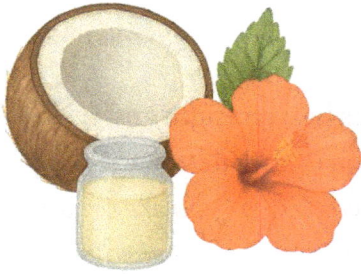

A rich mask that nourishes and restores shine. Coconut oil deeply conditions, while hibiscus petals support strong, soft strands. **Tip:** *Wrap your hair in a warm towel to boost absorption.*

Ingredients	Instructions
<ul><li>2 tbsp coconut oil (warmed to liquid)</li><li>1 tbsp dried hibiscus powder or crushed petals</li></ul>	1. Warm coconut oil gently until liquid. 2. Mix in hibiscus powder until smooth. 3. Apply to damp hair, focusing on ends. 4. Leave for 20–30 minutes, then rinse with mild shampoo.

Aloe Vera & Lemon Scalp Gel

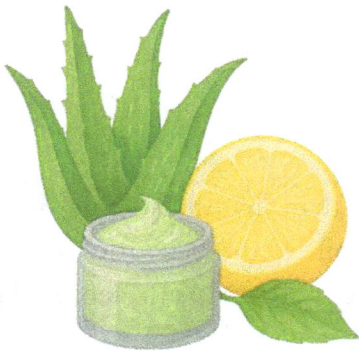

This cooling gel balances the scalp and helps reduce excess oil. Aloe soothes the skin, while lemon adds a refreshing cleanse.

Safety: *Avoid applying lemon juice on irritated or broken skin.*

Ingredients	Instructions
<ul><li>3 tbsp aloe vera gel</li><li>1 tsp fresh lemon juice</li><li>3 drops tea tree essential oil (optional)</li></ul>	1. Mix aloe gel with lemon juice in a small bowl. 2. Add tea tree oil if desired and blend well. 3. Apply directly to the scalp and massage gently. 4. Leave for 15 minutes, then rinse with lukewarm water.

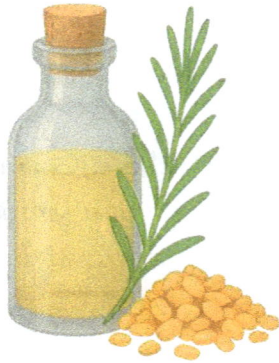

Fenugreek Seed Hair Strength Tonic

A nourishing tonic that improves hair strength and resilience. Fenugreek seeds release mucilage that hydrates the scalp and supports hair growth. **Safety:** *Avoid use if you are pregnant or taking blood-sugar medication without medical advice.*

Ingredients	Instructions
• 2 tbsp fenugreek seeds (soaked overnight) • 1 cup water	1. Soak fenugreek seeds in water overnight. 2. Blend the seeds with the soaking water until smooth. 3. Apply the mixture to scalp and roots. 4. Leave for 20 minutes, then rinse thoroughly.

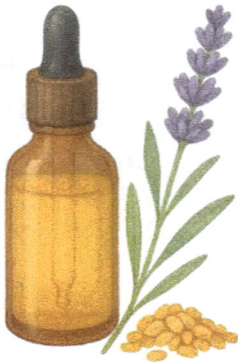

Lavender & Argan Oil Overnight Serum

A calming overnight serum that hydrates hair while promoting relaxation. Argan oil nourishes and softens strands, while lavender oil soothes both scalp and senses. **Tip:** *Use once a week for silky, manageable hair.*

Ingredients	Instructions
• 3 tbsp aloe vera gel • 1 tsp fresh lemon juice • 3 drops tea tree essential oil (optional)	1. Mix aloe gel with lemon juice in a small bowl. 2. Add tea tree oil if desired and blend well. 3. Apply directly to the scalp and massage gently. 4. Leave for 15 minutes, then rinse with lukewarm water.

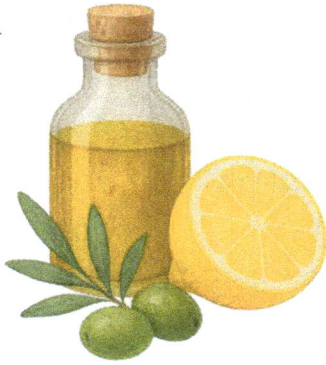

Olive Oil & Lemon Nail Soak

A simple soak that strengthens brittle nails and softens cuticles. Olive oil nourishes deeply, while lemon brightens and refreshes. **Safety**: *Avoid lemon on open cuts; use in the evening to prevent sun sensitivity.*

Ingredients	Instructions
<ul><li>2 tbsp olive oil (slightly warmed)</li><li>1 tsp fresh lemon juice</li><li>Small bowl</li></ul>	1. Warm olive oil gently until comfortable to touch. 2. Pour into a small bowl and add lemon juice. 3. Soak nails for 10–15 minutes. 4. Rinse and pat dry.

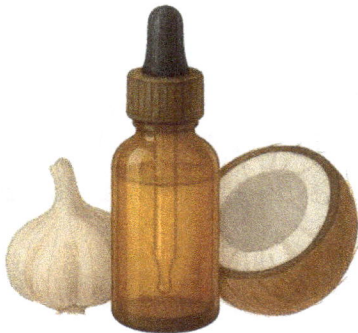

Garlic & Coconut Nail Serum

A strengthening serum that supports weak or splitting nails. Garlic's natural compounds reinforce nail structure, while coconut oil locks in moisture. **Safety:** *Test on one nail first, as garlic can cause skin sensitivity.*

Ingredients	Instructions
<ul><li>2 cloves garlic (crushed)</li><li>2 tbsp coconut oil (warmed to liquid)</li><li>Small glass jar</li></ul>	1. Crush garlic cloves and place them in a small jar. 2. Pour warm coconut oil over the garlic. 3. Let infuse for 24 hours, then strain. 4. Apply a drop to each nail and massage gently.

Horsetail & Rosemary Strengthening Tea

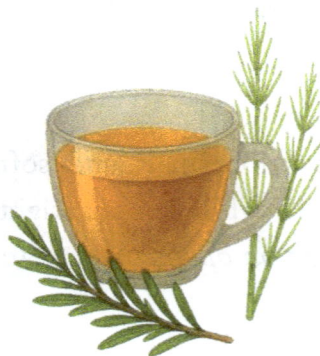

This mineral-rich tea supports both nail and hair health. Horsetail provides silica for resilience, while rosemary stimulates circulation for stronger growth. **Safety:** *Avoid horsetail during pregnancy or if you have kidney conditions.*

Ingredients	Instructions
• 1 tbsp dried horsetail • 1 tsp dried rosemary • 1 cup hot water	1. Place horsetail and rosemary in a teapot. 2. Pour hot water over them. 3. Cover and steep for 10 minutes. 4. Strain and drink warm.

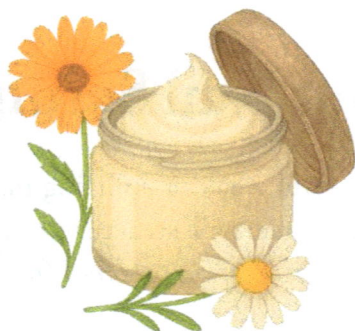

Calendula & Chamomile Hand Cream

A nourishing cream that soothes and protects dry hands. Calendula helps repair the skin barrier, while chamomile calms irritation. **Tip:** *Apply after washing hands or before bed to protect and soften skin.*

Ingredients	Instructions
• 2 tbsp calendula-infused oil • 1 tbsp shea butter • 1 tbsp beeswax • 1 tsp dried chamomile flowers (infused in the oil)	1. Melt beeswax and shea butter in a double boiler. 2. Stir in calendula-infused oil. 3. Strain if needed to remove chamomile pieces. 4. Pour into a small tin and let solidify.

Joints, Muscles & Inflammation Relief

S tiffness in the morning, sore muscles after exercise, or the dull ache that lingers in your joints can quietly shape the way you move through the day. Even small discomforts can make it harder to enjoy simple activities like walking, cooking, or sitting comfortably at your desk. When inflammation builds up, the body signals that it needs care and support.

The first instinct is often to ignore the pain or rely on quick over-the-counter solutions. But natural remedies can offer an accessible way to soothe discomfort while helping your body restore balance. With a few herbs, roots, and basic household items, you can create simple treatments that bring relief right where you need it.

In this chapter, you will explore practical recipes that focus on three key areas of support:

- **Herbal teas and infusions** that ease stiffness and calm inflammation from within. Ingredients such as turmeric, ginger, and nettle provide warmth, minerals, and natural comfort.

- **Decoctions, oils, and balms** that can be applied directly to sore muscles or joints, delivering soothing or warming effects through the skin.

- **Baths, compresses, and soaks** that combine water and herbs like rosemary, chamomile, or Epsom salts to relax muscles and ease tension after physical effort.

These remedies are quick to prepare and flexible enough to fit into daily life. You can brew a tea in a few minutes, prepare a simple poultice with dried herbs and warm water, or create a bath soak that transforms your evening routine into a moment of recovery. Many can also be made ahead and kept ready, so relief is always close at hand.

The aim of these recipes is to help you respond to discomfort in a calm, supportive way. They are not complicated treatments but practical options that let you care for your body naturally. By making them part of your routine, you can ease everyday aches, support joint health, and maintain mobility with greater ease.

Turmeric & Ginger Anti-Inflammatory Tea

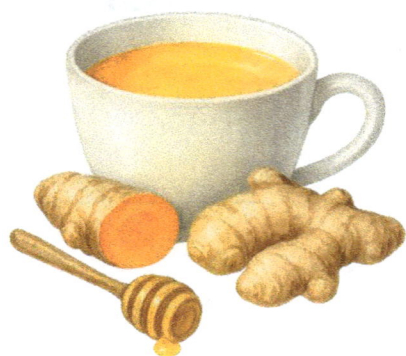

A warm, golden tea that soothes stiff joints and supports the body's natural anti-inflammatory response. Enjoy it in the morning or after physical activity to ease tension and bring comfort. **Tip**: *Add a tiny pinch of black pepper to enhance turmeric's absorption.*

Ingredients	Instructions
• 1 tsp grated fresh ginger • ½ tsp turmeric powder (or fresh grated root) • 1 cup hot water • 1 tsp honey (optional)	1. Place ginger and turmeric in a mug. 2. Pour hot water over the herbs. 3. Stir well, cover, and steep for 7–8 minutes. 4. Strain and add honey if desired.

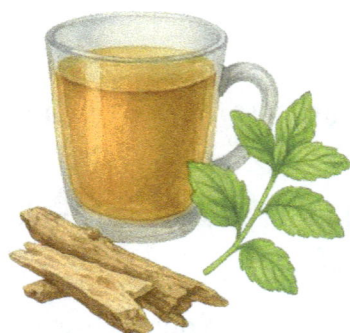

Willow Bark & Mint Infusion

A soothing herbal infusion that brings natural relief to aching joints. Willow bark offers traditional support for discomfort, while mint adds a cooling freshness to calm the body. **Safety:** Avoid willow bark if allergic to aspirin or taking blood-thinning medication.

Ingredients	Instructions
• 1 tsp dried willow bark • 1 tsp dried peppermint leaves • 1 cup hot water	1. Place willow bark in a small pot with water. 2. Simmer gently for 10 minutes. 3. Remove from heat, add peppermint, and cover for 5 minutes. 4. Strain and sip warm.

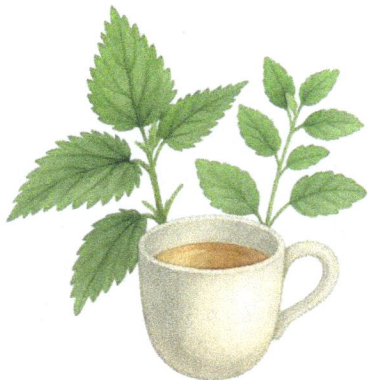

Nettle & Lemon Balm Comfort Tea

This mineral-rich blend eases muscle fatigue and soothes stiffness. Nettle nourishes with calcium and magnesium, while lemon balm relaxes both body and mind for gentle comfort.

Ingredients	Instructions
• 1 tbsp dried nettle leaves • 1 tsp dried lemon balm leaves • 1 cup hot water	1. Place nettle and lemon balm in a teapot. 2. Pour hot water and cover. 3. Steep for 8–10 minutes. 4. Strain and drink slowly.

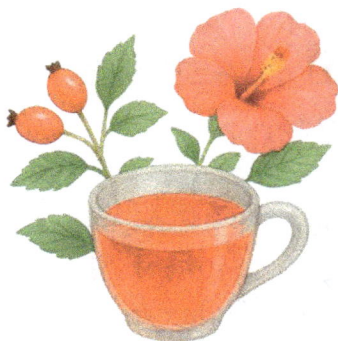

Rosehip & Hibiscus Anti-Inflammatory Brew

A vibrant red brew packed with vitamin C and antioxidants. Rosehip and hibiscus help calm mild inflammation while offering a tangy, refreshing flavor. **Tip:** *Add a spoonful of honey if you prefer a sweeter taste.*

Ingredients	Instructions
• 1 tbsp dried rosehips (crushed) • 1 tbsp dried hibiscus petals • 1 cup hot water	1. Place rosehips and hibiscus in a teapot. 2. Pour hot water over them and cover. 3. Steep for 10 minutes. 4. Strain and enjoy hot or chilled.

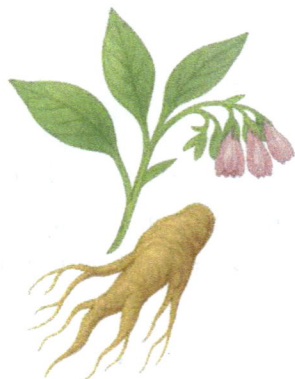

Comfrey Root Healing Poultice

A traditional remedy that soothes minor joint aches and helps support recovery from small strains or bumps. The moist, cooling paste can be applied directly to the affected area. **Safety**: *Avoid applying comfrey on broken skin or using it during pregnancy or breastfeeding.*

Ingredients	Instructions
• 2 tbsp dried comfrey root (powdered or crushed) • Warm water (enough to form a paste) • Clean cotton cloth	1. Mix comfrey root with enough warm water to form a thick paste. 2. Spread the paste onto a clean cloth. 3. Apply over the sore joint for 15–20 minutes.

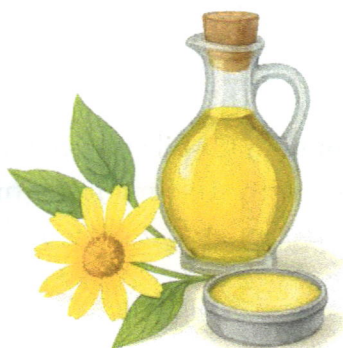

Arnica & Olive Oil Massage Balm

A soothing balm to ease tense muscles and sore spots. Arnica has long been valued for calming discomfort, while olive oil nourishes and softens the skin. **Safety**: *Do not apply arnica on broken skin or open wounds.*

Ingredients	Instructions
• 2 tbsp arnica-infused oil • 2 tbsp olive oil • 1 tbsp beeswax	1. Melt beeswax gently in a double boiler. 2. Stir in arnica-infused oil and olive oil. 3. Pour into a small jar or tin and let cool. 4. Massage onto sore muscles as needed.

Turmeric & Black Pepper Joint Paste

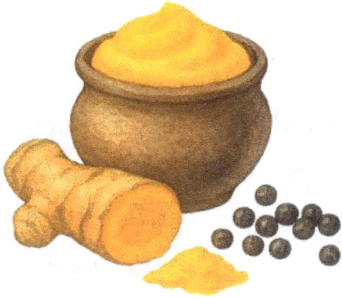

A simple paste for local application on stiff or swollen joints. Turmeric provides warmth and balance, while black pepper enhances its natural activity. **Safety**: *Test on a small skin area first; turmeric may stain. Avoid if using blood-thinning medication.*

Ingredients	Instructions
<ul><li>1 tbsp turmeric powder</li><li>½ tsp black pepper</li><li>2 tbsp warm coconut or olive oil</li></ul>	1. Mix turmeric and black pepper with the oil to form a smooth paste. 2. Apply directly to the affected joint. 3. Leave for 15–20 minutes, then rinse gently.

Ginger & Mustard Seed Warming Rub

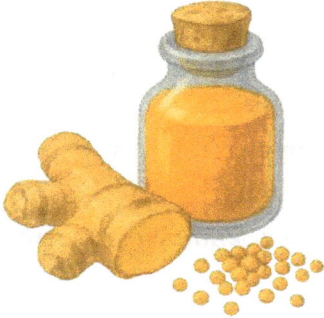

A warming rub that stimulates circulation and eases muscle stiffness. Ginger brings heat and comfort, while mustard seeds provide a gentle tingling effect that encourages flexibility. **Safety**: *Test on a small patch of skin first; discontinue if irritation occurs.*

Ingredients	Instructions
<ul><li>1 tbsp mustard seeds (crushed)</li><li>1 tsp fresh ginger juice</li><li>2 tbsp olive oil</li></ul>	1. Lightly crush mustard seeds. 2. Warm olive oil gently and stir in ginger juice and mustard seeds. 3. Massage the warm mixture onto stiff or sore areas.

Eucalyptus & Peppermint Cooling Gel

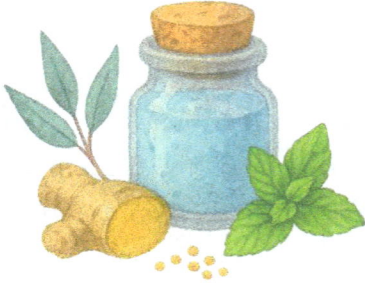

This refreshing gel soothes hot, tired muscles after activity. Eucalyptus eases tension, while peppermint cools and revives. Keep it in the fridge for an extra calming effect. **Safety**: *Avoid contact with eyes and mucous membranes; not recommended for young children.*

Ingredients	Instructions
<ul><li>2 tbsp aloe vera gel</li><li>1 tsp eucalyptus essential oil</li><li>1 tsp peppermint essential oil</li></ul>	1. Place aloe gel in a clean bowl. 2. Add essential oils and mix until smooth. 3. Transfer to a small jar and store in the fridge. 4. Apply a thin layer to tired muscles.

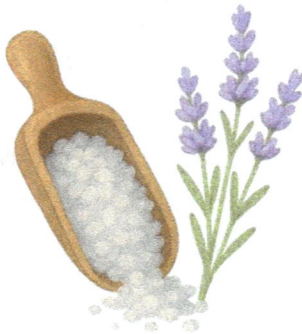

Epsom Salt & Lavender Bath

A deeply relaxing bath that melts away tension after intense physical effort. Epsom salt supports muscle relaxation, while lavender calms the senses. **Tip**: *Light a candle nearby to create an even more relaxing atmosphere.*

Ingredients	Instructions
<ul><li>1 cup Epsom salt</li><li>½ cup dried lavender flowers</li></ul>	<ul><li>Combine Epsom salt and lavender in a bowl.</li><li>Add the mixture to warm bathwater.</li><li>Stir gently and soak for 20 minutes.</li></ul>

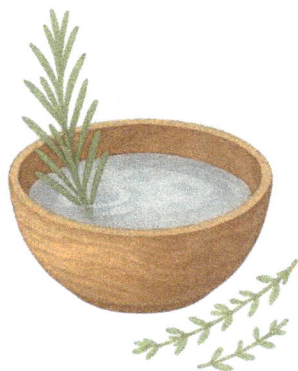

Rosemary & Thyme Foot Soak

A soothing soak that eases stiff joints and refreshes tired feet. Rosemary stimulates circulation, while thyme supports relaxation and comfort.

Ingredients	Instructions
<ul><li>1 tbsp dried rosemary</li><li>1 tbsp dried thyme</li><li>Basin of warm water</li></ul>	1. Place rosemary and thyme in a bowl or basin. 2. Pour warm water over the herbs. 3. Let steep for 5 minutes, then soak your feet for 15–20 minutes.

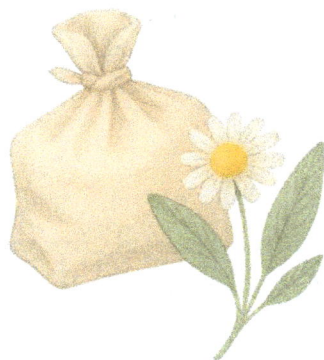

Chamomile & Sage Compress

This gentle compress calms localized tension and provides comfort to sore muscles. Chamomile soothes irritation, while sage offers a grounding herbal warmth. **Safety**: *Not recommended for people with known allergies to chamomile or sage.*

Ingredients	Instructions
<ul><li>2 tbsp dried chamomile flowers</li><li>1 tbsp dried sage leaves</li><li>2 cups hot water</li><li>Clean cotton cloth</li></ul>	1. Place chamomile and sage in a bowl. 2. Pour hot water over them and steep for 8 minutes. 3. Soak the cloth in the infusion, wring gently, and apply warm to the sore area.

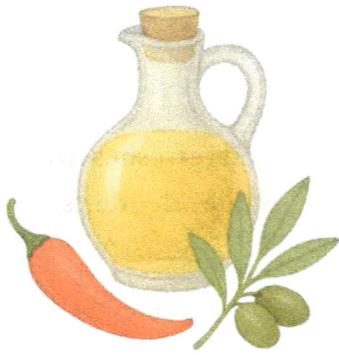

Cayenne & Olive Oil Warming Massage Oil

A stimulating massage oil that helps ease chronic stiffness and boost circulation. Cayenne creates gentle heat, while olive oil carries its warming effect deep into the muscles. **Safety**: *Always test on a small skin area first; avoid contact with eyes and sensitive skin.*

Ingredients	Instructions
<ul><li>1 tbsp cayenne pepper powder</li><li>½ cup olive oil</li><li>Small glass jar</li></ul>	1. Warm the olive oil gently. 2. Stir in cayenne powder until well blended. 3. Pour into a jar and let infuse for 24 hours. 4. Strain before applying to stiff joints or sore muscles.

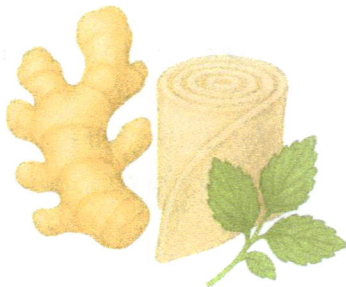

Ginger & Lemon Balm Warm Wrap

A comforting wrap for evening use when muscles feel tight and sore. Ginger stimulates warmth and circulation, while lemon balm adds a calming touch for relaxation. **Tip**: *Rewarm the cloth in hot infusion if it cools too quickly.*

Ingredients	Instructions
<ul><li>2 tbsp fresh ginger slices</li><li>1 tbsp dried lemon balm leaves</li><li>2 cups hot water</li><li>Clean cotton cloth or towel</li></ul>	1. Place ginger and lemon balm in a bowl. 2. Pour hot water and steep for 8–10 minutes. 3. Soak a clean cloth in the infusion, wring gently, and apply to sore muscles. 4. Leave on for 15–20 minutes.

Respiratory, Sinus & Allergy Relief

Clear breathing is something you rarely think about until it becomes difficult. A sudden change in weather can leave you with a blocked nose. A long day in dusty air might irritate your throat. Seasonal pollen can trigger sneezing fits that interrupt your focus. When your respiratory system feels heavy or congested, even simple tasks like climbing stairs or having a conversation can seem harder than they should.

In these situations, natural remedies can offer practical and immediate support. You do not need to wait for an appointment or reach for strong medication unless necessary. A few herbs, flowers, or pantry items can quickly transform into steams, gargles, or drinks that help you feel more at ease.

Here are some common scenarios and the types of remedies you will find useful in this chapter:

- **Mild coughs and sore throats** – Honey, thyme, or licorice root can be prepared into teas or syrups that coat the throat and ease irritation.

- **Nasal congestion and sinus pressure** – Peppermint, eucalyptus, or rosemary can be added to hot water for a steam that opens your airways and clears your head.

- **Seasonal allergies** – Herbs like nettle and elderflower provide gentle support when pollen makes breathing uncomfortable.

- **Everyday refreshment** – Simple sprays or gargles with ingredients such as chamomile, lemon, or salt can be prepared in minutes and used throughout the day.

These remedies are designed to be straightforward and convenient. Most require nothing more than hot water, a bowl, or a jar. You can prepare a steam in the kitchen, a throat gargle in the bathroom, or a calming tea before bed. Many of the ingredients are already familiar, which makes it easy to integrate them into your routine without extra effort.

The recipes that follow are not meant to replace medical treatment in serious cases, but they can serve as your first line of support when your nose feels blocked, your throat is sore, or seasonal changes affect your breathing. By keeping a few of these simple preparations ready, you give yourself quick and natural ways to breathe easier and stay comfortable in daily life.

Thyme & Honey Lung Support Tea

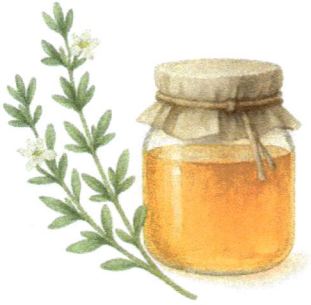

This warm tea gently calms persistent coughs and supports clearer, more comfortable breathing. Thyme helps open the chest, while honey soothes irritation in the throat. Sip it slowly in the evening or after a day exposed to cold air to relax your lungs. **Tip**: Drink 2–3 times daily to ease coughs.

Ingredients	Instructions
• 1 tsp dried thyme • 1 tsp raw honey • 1 cup hot water	1. Place thyme in a mug and pour hot water over it. 2. Cover and steep for 7 minutes. 3. Strain and stir in honey before sipping warm.

Peppermint & Eucalyptus Clear Breathing Tea

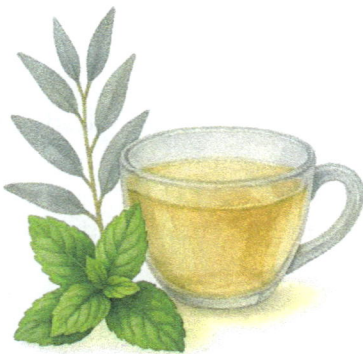

This refreshing tea clears blocked sinuses and eases nasal congestion with every sip. Peppermint provides a cooling lift, while eucalyptus gently opens your airways. Keep a warm thermos on hand during the day when you need to breathe more freely. **Safety**: *Avoid eucalyptus for children under 2 years.*

Ingredients	Instructions
• 1 tsp dried peppermint leaves • 1 drop eucalyptus oil (food grade) or 1 tsp dried eucalyptus leaves • 1 cup hot water	1. Add peppermint and eucalyptus to a cup. 2. Pour hot water over the herbs. 3. Cover, steep for 6–7 minutes, strain, and sip slowly.

Ginger & Licorice Root Comfort Infusion

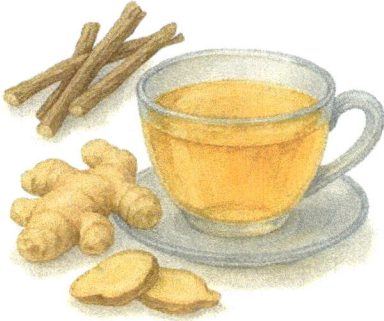

A soothing infusion that eases dry, scratchy throats and calms irritated airways. Ginger warms from within, while licorice coats the throat, bringing lasting relief. Enjoy it after being outdoors in cold, dry air or when your voice feels strained. **Safety**: *Avoid licorice if you have high blood pressure.*

Ingredients	Instructions
• 1 tsp fresh ginger slices • 1 tsp dried licorice root • 1 cup water	1. Place ginger and licorice in a small pot with water. 2. Simmer gently for 10 minutes. 3. Strain and sip warm.

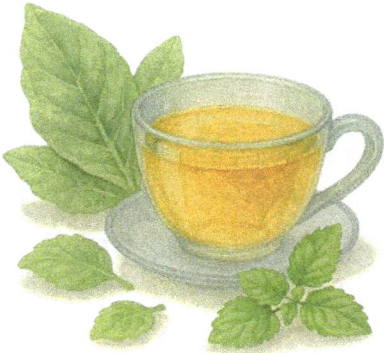

Mullein Leaf & Lemon Balm Tea

This gentle tea supports lung health and encourages smooth, easy breathing. Mullein softens irritated airways, while lemon balm brings calm to both body and mind. Drink it warm during seasonal changes or when you feel chest tightness.

Ingredients	Instructions
• 1 tbsp dried mullein leaves • 1 tsp dried lemon balm leaves • 1 cup hot water	1. Combine mullein and lemon balm in a teapot. 2. Pour hot water and cover. 3. Steep 10 minutes, strain carefully, and drink warm.

Nettle & Elderflower Allergy Tea

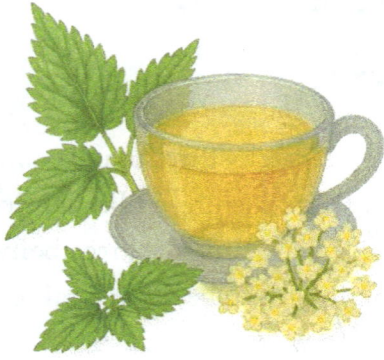

This herbal tea helps ease seasonal allergies by calming sensitivity and supporting the respiratory system. Nettle provides natural minerals that strengthen resilience, while elderflower soothes sinus irritation. Enjoy a cup daily during spring or high-pollen days.

Ingredients	Instructions
• 1 tbsp dried nettle leaves • 1 tbsp dried elderflowers • 1 cup hot water	1. Add nettle and elderflowers to a teapot. 2. Pour hot water over them and cover. 3. Steep 8–10 minutes, strain, and enjoy warm.

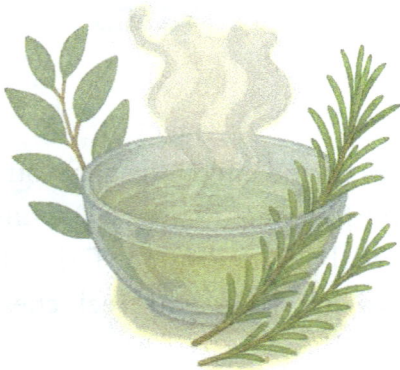

Eucalyptus & Rosemary Steam Inhalation

A fragrant steam that helps clear sinuses and open blocked nasal passages. Eucalyptus supports free breathing, while rosemary stimulates circulation and brings a refreshing aroma. Use this steam when congestion makes it hard to breathe deeply. **Tip**: *Keep your eyes closed to prevent irritation from the steam.*

Ingredients	Instructions
• 1 tbsp dried eucalyptus leaves • 1 tbsp dried rosemary • 3 cups hot water • Towel	1. Place herbs in a large bowl. 2. Pour hot water over them. 3. Lean over with a towel over your head and inhale deeply for 5–10 minutes.

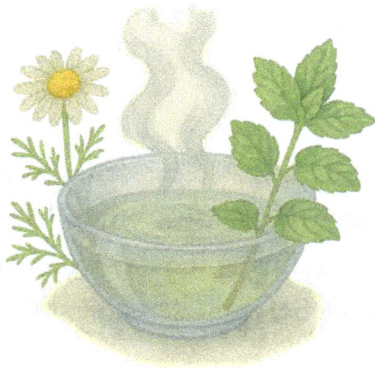

Chamomile & Peppermint Steam Bowl

This gentle steam relaxes the body while soothing congestion and easing nasal pressure. Chamomile calms the sinuses, and peppermint clears blocked passages with its cooling vapor. Perfect for a comforting evening ritual when your head feels heavy.

Ingredients	Instructions
<ul><li>1 tbsp dried chamomile flowers</li><li>1 tbsp dried peppermint leaves</li><li>3 cups hot water</li><li>Towel</li></ul>	1. Place chamomile and peppermint in a bowl. 2. Pour hot water over them. 3. Lean over, cover your head with a towel, and inhale for 5–10 minutes.

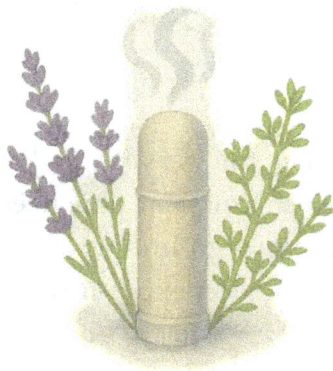

Lavender & Thyme Inhaler

A portable inhaler for quick, natural relief from a blocked nose. Lavender offers a soothing floral calm, while thyme clears the airways with its herbal freshness. Keep it in your bag for instant comfort while traveling or on the go. **Safety:** *Essential oils are strong—avoid use for children under 6 years.*

Ingredients	Instructions
<ul><li>5 drops lavender essential oil</li><li>5 drops thyme essential oil</li><li>1 cotton wick or pad</li><li>1 small inhaler tube</li></ul>	1. Insert the cotton wick into the inhaler tube. 2. Add the essential oils to the wick. 3. Inhale through the tube when congestion strikes.

Peppermint & Lemon Nasal Spray

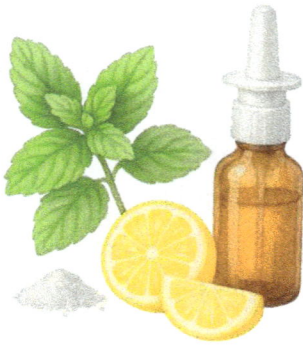

This light spray refreshes and helps clear mild nasal congestion. Peppermint sharpens the senses, while lemon adds a clean, uplifting scent. Use it during the day when you feel blocked and need a quick reset. **Safety:** *Use sparingly; not suitable for children under 6.*

Ingredients	Instructions
• ½ cup distilled water • ¼ tsp sea salt • 1 drop peppermint essential oil • 2 drops lemon essential oil	1. Mix water and sea salt in a small spray bottle. 2. Add the essential oils and shake gently. 3. Spray lightly into nostrils as needed.

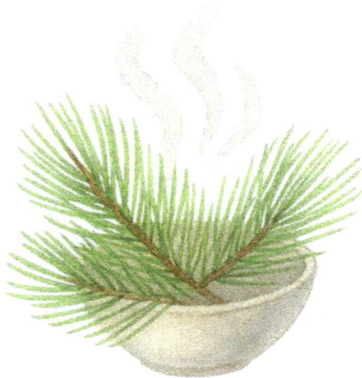

Pine Needle Steam for Seasonal Relief

A purifying steam that helps open the airways and ease seasonal congestion. The forest-fresh aroma of pine needles supports clearer breathing and brings a grounding sense of renewal. Ideal during allergy season or after exposure to cold, damp weather.

Ingredients	Instructions
• 1 tbsp fresh or dried pine needles • 3 cups hot water • Towel	1. Place pine needles in a large bowl. 2. Pour hot water over them. 3. Cover your head with a towel and inhale deeply for 5–10 minutes.

Honey & Ginger Cough Syrup

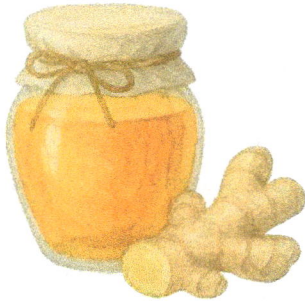

This homemade syrup eases throat irritation and reduces persistent coughing. Honey coats and soothes, while ginger adds warmth and comfort. Take a spoonful in the morning or before bed to keep coughing under control.

Ingredients	Instructions
• ½ cup raw honey 2 tbsp fresh ginger juice or grated ginger	1. Warm honey gently in a small saucepan. 2. Stir in ginger juice until blended. 3. Store in a clean jar and take 1 tsp as needed.

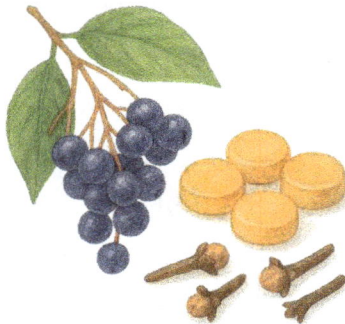

Elderberry & Clove Throat Lozenges

These homemade lozenges bring comfort to a sore or irritated throat. Elderberry provides protective support, while clove adds gentle warmth and a soothing flavor. Keep them in your bag for quick relief during cold season.

Safety: *Not suitable for children under 2 years.*

Ingredients	Instructions
• ½ cup elderberry syrup • 1 tbsp honey • ½ tsp ground cloves • ½ cup sugar (optional, for hard texture)	1. Simmer elderberry syrup, honey, and cloves until thick. 2. Drop small spoonfuls onto parchment paper. 3. Let harden into lozenges and store in a jar.

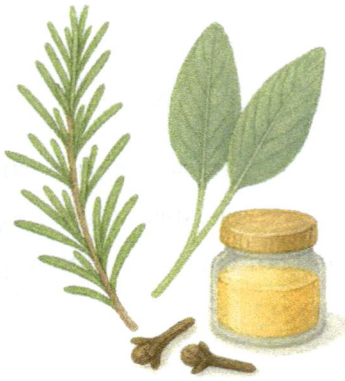

Rosemary & Sage Chest Rub

This aromatic balm helps clear the chest and ease breathing during congestion. Rosemary stimulates circulation and opens airways, while sage adds a grounding herbal warmth. Massage onto the chest before bedtime to support restful sleep.

Ingredients	Instructions
<ul><li>2 tbsp olive oil</li><li>1 tbsp dried rosemary or 5 drops essential oil</li><li>1 tbsp dried sage or 5 drops essential oil</li><li>1 tbsp beeswax</li></ul>	1. Melt beeswax and olive oil in a double boiler. 2. Stir in rosemary and sage. 3. Pour into a small jar and let cool. 4. Rub gently on the chest before bed.

Chamomile & Salt Gargle

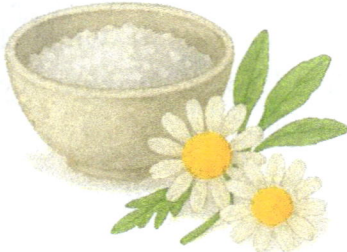

A simple yet effective rinse that soothes sore or irritated throats. Chamomile calms inflammation, while salt helps cleanse and reduce discomfort. Use after talking, singing, or during seasonal throat strain for fast relief.

Ingredients	Instructions
<ul><li>1 tsp dried chamomile flowers</li><li>½ tsp sea salt</li><li>1 cup hot water</li></ul>	1. Brew chamomile in hot water for 7 minutes. 2. Strain and let cool slightly. 3. Stir in salt and gargle for 30 seconds, repeating as needed.

Heart, Circulation & Healthy Blood Pressure

Your heart and circulatory system work silently every day to keep your body nourished and energized. A steady heartbeat, clear blood flow, and balanced pressure allow every cell to receive oxygen and nutrients. Yet stress, irregular sleep, heavy meals, and a lack of movement can place extra strain on this vital system. Over time, even mild imbalances may show up as fatigue, tension, or difficulty relaxing.

Caring for your heart does not have to mean complicated routines. Small daily choices can make a real difference. Natural remedies, prepared with common herbs and foods, provide a practical way to support circulation and maintain balance. They can also add comfort when you feel tense or when your body needs a gentle reset.

In this chapter, you will discover:

- **Teas and infusions** that encourage calm and steady circulation with ingredients such as hawthorn, linden, hibiscus, and lavender.

- **Tonics and drinks** that warm and stimulate, using ginger, cacao, garlic, or beets to keep blood moving and energy levels stable.

- **Practical supports** like broths or relaxing baths that combine nourishment and relaxation, easing pressure while calming the nervous system.

Most recipes are quick to prepare. A handful of dried blossoms can steep into a calming tea that encourages relaxation. A fresh juice with beet or pomegranate can give your circulation a natural boost. A simple herbal bath can lower tension at the end of a demanding day. Each remedy is designed to be accessible, enjoyable, and adaptable to your routine.

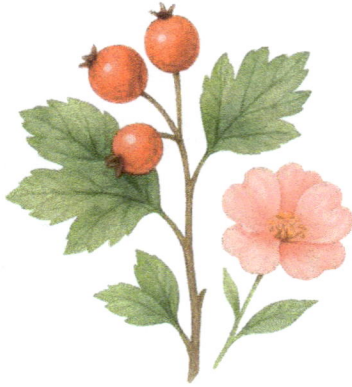

Hawthorn Berry & Rose Tea

A gentle tea that supports heart vitality and emotional well-being. Hawthorn berries strengthen circulation, while rose petals bring a soothing floral lift to both body and mood.

Safety: *Hawthorn may interact with heart medications, consult your doctor if you are under treatment.*

Ingredients	Instructions
• 1 tbsp dried hawthorn berries • 1 tsp dried rose petals • 1 cup hot water	1. Place hawthorn berries in a small pot with water. 2. Simmer gently for 10 minutes. 3. Remove from heat, add rose petals, cover, and steep for 5 minutes. 4. Strain and sip warm.

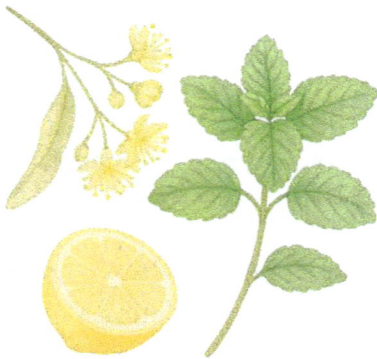

Linden Blossom & Lemon Balm Infusion

This calming infusion relaxes both body and mind, easing tension while gently supporting the heart. Perfect for winding down in the evening or during moments of restlessness.

Ingredients	Instructions
• 1 tbsp dried linden blossoms • 1 tsp dried lemon balm leaves • 1 cup hot water	1. Place linden and lemon balm in a teapot. 2. Pour hot water over them and cover. 3. Steep for 8–10 minutes. 4. Strain and enjoy warm.

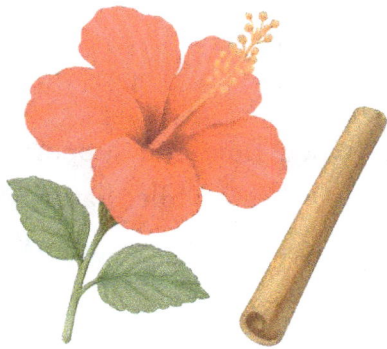

Hibiscus & Cinnamon Heart Tea

Bright and tangy hibiscus blends with warming cinnamon to support healthy blood pressure and circulation. A colorful tea that's both refreshing and comforting. **Safety**: *Avoid hibiscus if you have very low blood pressure or are pregnant, unless advised by a healthcare professional.*

Ingredients	Instructions
• 1 tbsp dried hibiscus petals • 1 small cinnamon stick or ½ tsp ground cinnamon • 1 cup hot water	1. Place hibiscus and cinnamon in a teapot. 2. Pour hot water over them and cover. 3. Steep for 7–8 minutes. 4. Strain and drink warm or chilled.

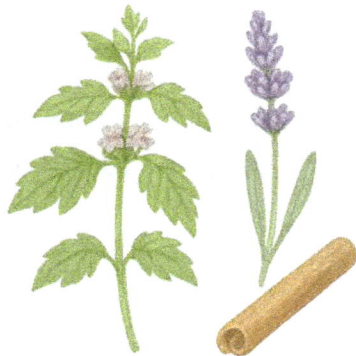

Motherwort & Lavender Tea

A grounding blend that steadies the heart and encourages emotional calm. Motherwort relaxes the nervous system, while lavender eases tension for a balanced state. **Safety**: *Avoid motherwort during pregnancy unless recommended by a healthcare professional.*

Ingredients	Instructions
• 1 tsp dried motherwort • 1 tsp dried lavender flowers • 1 cup hot water	1. Place motherwort and lavender in a cup. 2. Pour hot water and cover. 3. Steep for 7–8 minutes. 4. Strain and sip slowly.

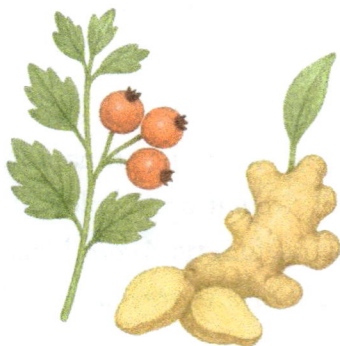

Hawthorn & Ginger Circulation Tonic

This warming tonic stimulates blood flow and supports a strong heart. Ginger adds gentle heat while hawthorn encourages healthy circulation. **Tip**: *Drink before a walk or light exercise to enhance circulation.*

Ingredients	Instructions
• 1 tbsp dried hawthorn berries • 1 tsp fresh ginger slices • 2 cups water	1. Place hawthorn and ginger in a pot with water. 2. Simmer gently for 15 minutes. 3. Strain and enjoy warm.

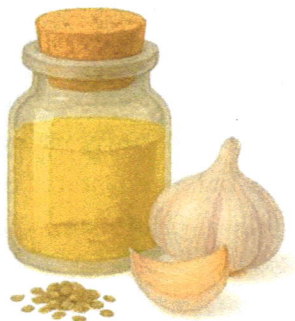

Garlic & Olive Oil Heart Tonic

A traditional remedy that nourishes the cardiovascular system. Garlic supports heart health, while olive oil provides healthy fats that protect vessels. **Safety**: *Avoid large amounts of garlic before surgery or if using blood-thinning medication.*

Ingredients	Instructions
• 2 cloves garlic (crushed) • 3 tbsp extra virgin olive oil • Small glass jar	1. Place crushed garlic in a clean jar. 2. Cover with olive oil and stir gently. 3. Let infuse for 12–24 hours. 4. Strain and store in a sealed container. 5. Take 1 tsp daily with meals.

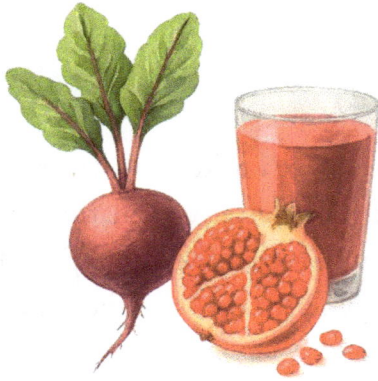

Beet & Pomegranate Vitality Juice

Rich in antioxidants and natural nitrates, this vibrant juice supports energy and healthy circulation. A refreshing option to enjoy in the morning or before exercise.

Ingredients	Instructions
• 1 medium beet (peeled and chopped) • ½ cup pomegranate seeds • 1 cup water	1. Place beet, pomegranate seeds, and water in a blender. 2. Blend until smooth. 3. Strain if desired and serve chilled.

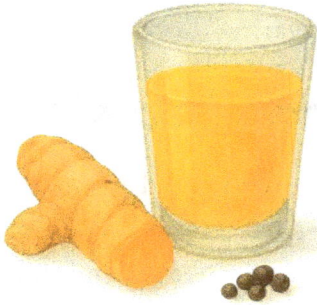

Turmeric & Black Pepper Golden Shot

A small yet powerful shot that helps support circulation and overall vitality. Turmeric offers antioxidant benefits, while black pepper boosts absorption. **Safety**: *Avoid high doses of turmeric if you are on blood-thinning medication.*

Ingredients	Instructions
• ½ tsp turmeric powder (or fresh grated turmeric) • 1 pinch black pepper • ½ cup warm water • 1 tsp honey (optional)	1. Add turmeric and black pepper to warm water. 2. Stir well until blended. 3. Add honey if desired and drink immediately.

Cacao & Cayenne Warming Drink

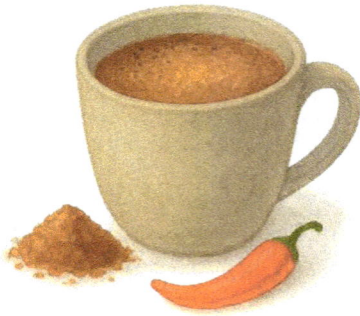

This bold drink blends rich cacao with a kick of cayenne pepper, warming the body and stimulating circulation. A comforting option on cold days when you need energy and focus. **Tip**: *Start with a very small pinch of cayenne and adjust to your taste.*

Ingredients	Instructions
• 1 cup warm milk or plant-based milk • 1 tsp raw cacao powder • 1 pinch cayenne pepper • 1 tsp honey or maple syrup (optional)	1. Warm the milk in a small pot. 2. Whisk in cacao and cayenne until smooth. 3. Sweeten with honey or maple syrup if desired. 4. Sip slowly while warm.

Celery Seed & Lemon Infusion

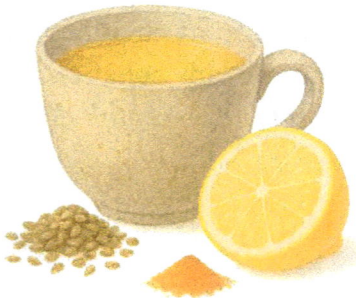

A light and refreshing tea that supports fluid balance and helps maintain steady blood pressure. Celery seeds offer natural diuretic qualities, while lemon brightens and uplifts. **Safety**: *Avoid celery seeds during pregnancy or if you have kidney disorders unless advised by a healthcare professional.*

Ingredients	Instructions
• 1 tsp celery seeds (lightly crushed) • 1 slice fresh lemon • 1 cup hot water	1. Place celery seeds in a cup. 2. Pour hot water over them and cover. 3. Steep for 10 minutes. 4. Add lemon slice, then sip slowly.

Hibiscus & Rosehip Cooling Drink

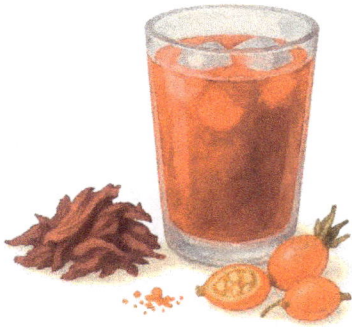

A tangy, refreshing drink that supports healthy blood pressure. Hibiscus offers circulatory balance, while rosehip adds a vitamin C boost and a bright flavor. **Safety**: *Avoid hibiscus during pregnancy or if you have very low blood pressure.*

Ingredients	Instructions
<ul><li>1 tbsp dried hibiscus petals</li><li>1 tbsp dried rosehips (crushed)</li><li>1 cup cold water</li><li>Ice cubes (optional)</li></ul>	1. Place hibiscus and rosehips in a cup or jar. 2. Pour cold water over the herbs. 3. Let steep for 15–20 minutes. 4. Strain, add ice if desired, and enjoy chilled.

Garlic & Parsley Heart-Healthy Broth

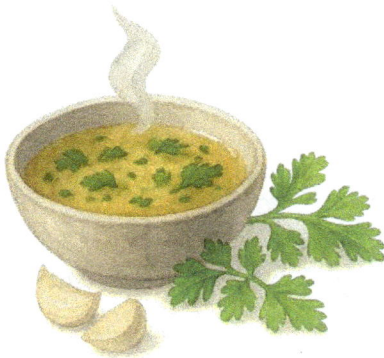

This nourishing broth combines garlic's traditional heart-supporting qualities with parsley's fresh minerals for circulation. A comforting way to warm up while caring for your cardiovascular health. **Safety**: *Limit garlic if taking blood-thinning medication.*

Ingredients	Instructions
<ul><li>3 cups water</li><li>3 garlic cloves (sliced)</li><li>2 tbsp fresh parsley (chopped)</li></ul>	1. Place garlic and water in a small pot. 2. Simmer for 15 minutes. 3. Add parsley and steep for 5 minutes. 4. Strain and sip warm.

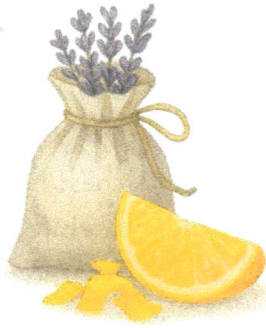

Lavender & Orange Relaxing Bath

A soothing bath that calms the senses and eases stress, indirectly supporting healthy blood pressure. Lavender promotes relaxation, while orange peel adds a bright, uplifting aroma.

Ingredients	Instructions
• ½ cup dried lavender flowers • Zest of 1 orange • 1 muslin bag or clean cotton cloth • Warm bathwater	1. Place lavender and orange zest in a muslin bag. 2. Tie securely and place in warm bathwater. 3. Let steep for 5 minutes. 4. Soak for 20 minutes, breathing deeply.

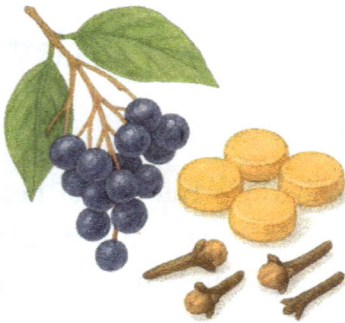

Ginkgo & Lemon Zest Circulation Tea

This light, uplifting tea supports healthy blood flow and mental alertness. Ginkgo leaves promote circulation to the brain and extremities, while lemon zest adds brightness and a refreshing note to each sip. **Safety**: *Ginkgo may interact with blood-thinning medication—consult your healthcare provider before use.*

Ingredients	Instructions
• 1 tsp dried ginkgo leaves • Zest of ½ fresh lemon • 1 cup hot water	1. Place ginkgo leaves and lemon zest in a teapot. 2. Pour hot water over the herbs. 3. Cover and steep for 8–10 minutes. 4. Strain and sip warm.

Urinary Tract & Kidney Comfort

The kidneys and urinary tract are responsible for filtering waste, balancing fluids, and keeping your body's internal system clear. When they are under stress, you may feel heaviness, bloating, or irritation that makes everyday activities more difficult. Instead of waiting for discomfort to intensify, you can support these organs with simple, natural remedies that are easy to prepare at home.

The recipes in this chapter are designed to be practical and accessible. They use ingredients you can find in a kitchen or local store, and they can be prepared in just a few steps. Each option focuses on keeping your system comfortable, hydrated, and balanced.

Here are some of the ways these remedies can help you:

- **Daily hydration support:** Light teas with nettle or dandelion encourage natural cleansing, while cucumber or parsley waters refresh and keep you hydrated.

- **Relief for irritation:** Cornsilk and chamomile ease bladder sensitivity, while marshmallow root offers a soothing, protective effect.

- **Cleansing and lightness:** Barley water with lemon or juniper with fennel helps the body release excess fluids and reduces bloating.

- **Mineral nourishment:** Herbs such as nettle, parsley, and hibiscus provide minerals that sustain kidney health while adding gentle flavor.

- **External comfort:** Simple sitz baths with calendula and chamomile or herbal steams with lemon zest and parsley bring soothing relief from the outside.

You do not need advanced tools to use these preparations. A mug, a pot of hot water, or a clean bowl is usually enough. Many remedies can be made in minutes and even kept on hand for later. Sipping a warm tea after meals, carrying an infused water during the day, or taking a short evening soak are practical ways to make this support part of your life.

These recipes are not medical treatments but reliable, natural tools that complement daily care. By choosing even one or two and using them consistently, you can reduce discomfort, support kidney function, and maintain a steady sense of inner balance.

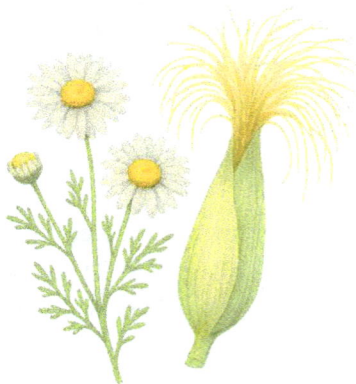

Cornsilk & Chamomile Soothing Tea

A gentle tea that calms irritation and supports urinary comfort. Cornsilk eases inflammation while chamomile relaxes the body, making it ideal during moments of bladder sensitivity. **Tip**: *Drink up to twice daily for gentle support.*

Ingredients	Instructions
• 1 tbsp dried cornsilk • 1 tsp dried chamomile flowers • 1 cup hot water	1. Place cornsilk and chamomile in a cup. 2. Pour hot water over the herbs. 3. Cover, steep for 8–10 minutes, then strain and sip warm.

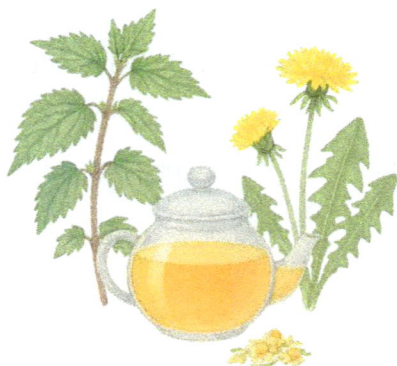

Nettle & Dandelion Leaf Tea

This mineral-rich infusion supports kidney function and helps the body eliminate excess fluids naturally. Perfect as a light daily tea to encourage gentle detox. **Safety**: *Avoid dandelion if allergic to ragweed family plants.*

Ingredients	Instructions
• 1 tbsp dried nettle leaves • 1 tbsp dried dandelion leaves • 1 cup hot water	1. Add nettle and dandelion leaves to a teapot. 2. Pour hot water over them and cover. 3. Steep for 10 minutes, strain, and enjoy warm.

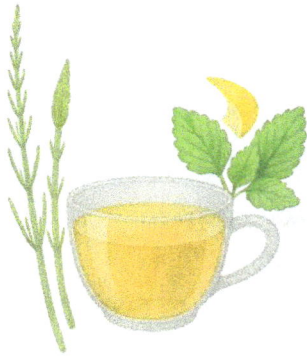

Horsetail & Lemon Balm Infusion

Horsetail provides natural silica that supports kidney and urinary health, while lemon balm brings a calming effect to ease tension. A soothing blend for promoting fluid balance. **Safety:** *Avoid horsetail if pregnant or dealing with kidney conditions.*

Ingredients	Instructions
• 1 tbsp dried horsetail • 1 tsp dried lemon balm leaves • 1 cup hot water	1. Place horsetail and lemon balm in a cup. 2. Pour hot water over the herbs. 3. Cover and steep for 8–10 minutes, then strain.

Parsley & Peppermint Tea

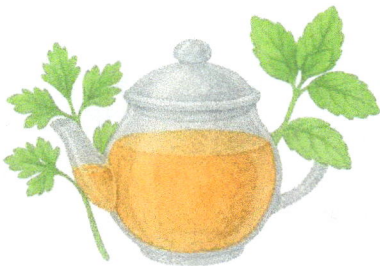

A light, refreshing tea that helps cool the body and support natural fluid elimination. Parsley encourages urinary flow, while peppermint adds a soothing, fresh lift. **Safety:** *Avoid large amounts of parsley during pregnancy.*

Ingredients	Instructions
• 1 tbsp fresh parsley leaves (chopped) • 1 tsp dried peppermint leaves • 1 cup hot water	1. Place parsley and peppermint in a teapot. 2. Pour hot water and cover. 3. Steep for 7–8 minutes, strain, and sip warm or cooled.

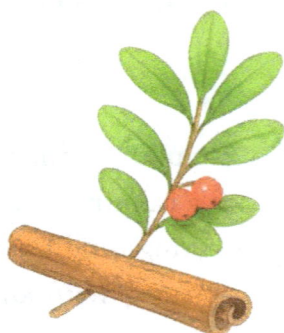

Uva Ursi & Cinnamon Decoction

Traditionally valued for urinary comfort, uva ursi supports bladder health, while cinnamon adds warmth and flavor. A grounding option during mild urinary discomfort. **Safety**: *Avoid uva ursi during pregnancy or long-term use; consult a healthcare professional before trying.*

Ingredients	Instructions
<ul><li>1 tbsp dried uva ursi leaves</li><li>1 small cinnamon stick</li><li>2 cups water</li></ul>	1. Place uva ursi and cinnamon in a pot with water. 2. Simmer gently for 15 minutes. 3. Strain and sip warm.

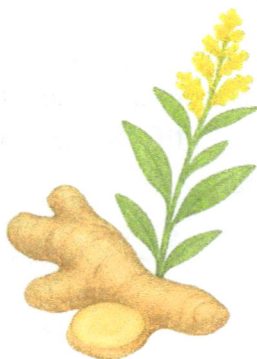

Goldenrod & Ginger Kidney Tonic

Goldenrod supports kidney function and urinary flow, while ginger adds gentle warmth to ease discomfort. A simple tonic to enjoy when you feel heavy or sluggish. **Safety**: *Avoid goldenrod if you have severe kidney disease or known allergies to related plants.*

Ingredients	Instructions
<ul><li>1 tbsp dried goldenrod</li><li>1 tsp fresh ginger slices</li><li>1 cup hot water</li></ul>	1. Place goldenrod and ginger in a teapot. 2. Pour hot water and cover. 3. Steep for 8–10 minutes, strain, and sip warm.

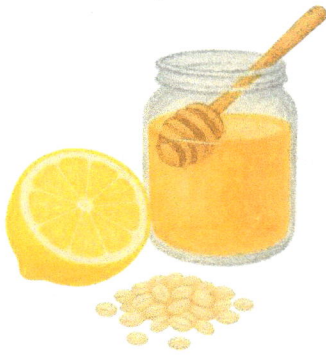

Barley Water with Lemon & Honey

This classic drink hydrates the body and gently soothes the bladder. Barley supports cleansing, while lemon and honey add lightness and comfort. **Tip**: *Store in the fridge for up to 2 days and sip throughout the day.*

Ingredients	Instructions
• 2 tbsp pearl barley • 2 cups water • 1 tsp honey (optional) • Juice of ½ fresh lemon	1. Rinse barley under running water. 2. Place in a pot with water and simmer for 20 minutes. 3. Strain, let cool slightly, then stir in lemon juice and honey. 4. Drink warm or chilled.

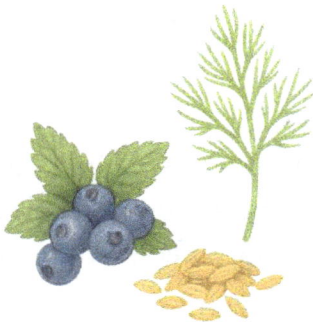

Juniper Berry & Fennel Decoction

A gently cleansing drink that supports kidney health and digestion. Juniper berries promote urinary flow, while fennel soothes bloating and adds a mild sweetness. **Safety**: *Avoid juniper berries during pregnancy or if you have kidney disease.*

Ingredients	Instructions
• 1 tbsp dried juniper berries (crushed) • 1 tsp fennel seeds 2 cups water	1. Place juniper berries and fennel in a small pot with water. 2. Simmer gently for 12–15 minutes. 3. Strain and drink warm.

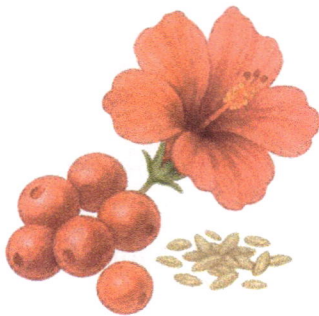

Cranberry & Hibiscus Refreshing Drink

A tart, ruby-colored drink that helps support urinary tract health and hydration. Cranberry is known for its protective qualities, while hibiscus adds a refreshing tang and extra antioxidants. **Safety**: *Avoid large amounts of cranberry if you are prone to kidney stones.*

Ingredients	Instructions
<ul><li>½ cup fresh or dried cranberries</li><li>1 tbsp dried hibiscus petals</li><li>2 cups water</li><li>Honey or maple syrup (optional)</li></ul>	1. Simmer cranberries in water for 10 minutes. 2. Add hibiscus, cover, and steep for 5–7 minutes. 3. Strain and sweeten to taste. 4. Serve warm or chilled.

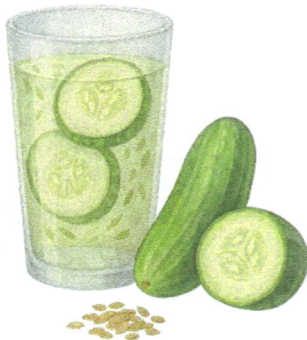

Celery Seed & Cucumber Infused Water

This crisp infusion hydrates and encourages natural detox. Celery seeds act as a gentle diuretic, while cucumber cools and refreshes, making it a perfect all-day sip. **Safety**: *Avoid celery seeds during pregnancy or if you have kidney disorders unless advised by a doctor.*

Ingredients	Instructions
<ul><li>1 tsp celery seeds (lightly crushed)</li><li>½ cucumber (sliced)</li><li>2 cups cold water</li></ul>	1. Place celery seeds and cucumber slices in a large jar. 2. Pour cold water over them. 3. Let infuse for 20–30 minutes before drinking.

Pumpkin Seed & Mint Snack Mix

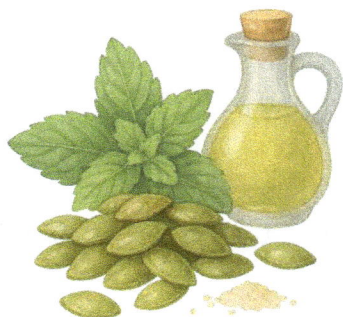

This crunchy mix supports urinary well-being and provides essential minerals like zinc and magnesium. Pumpkin seeds nourish the urinary system, while mint leaves add a refreshing flavor. **Tip**: *Store in an airtight container for a quick, mineral-rich snack.*

Ingredients	Instructions
<ul><li>½ cup pumpkin seeds (lightly toasted)</li><li>1 tbsp dried mint leaves</li><li>1 tsp olive oil</li><li>A pinch of sea salt</li></ul>	1. Toss pumpkin seeds with olive oil and mint leaves. 2. Spread on a baking sheet and toast lightly at low heat for 5–7 minutes. 3. Sprinkle with sea salt and let cool before enjoying.

Warm Sitz Bath with Chamomile & Calendula

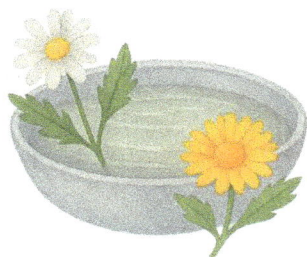

A gentle sitz bath that eases pelvic tension and soothes urinary discomfort. Chamomile calms irritation, while calendula supports skin comfort and healing. **Safety**: *Not recommended for use during pregnancy without medical advice.*

Ingredients	Instructions
<ul><li>2 tbsp dried chamomile flowers</li><li>2 tbsp dried calendula petals</li></ul>Basin of warm water	1. Fill a basin with warm water deep enough to sit comfortably. 2. Add chamomile and calendula. 3. Let steep for 5 minutes, then sit and soak for 15–20 minutes.

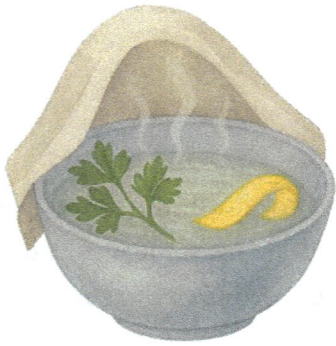

Parsley & Lemon Herbal Steam

This fragrant steam supports urinary comfort from the outside. Parsley helps stimulate natural cleansing, while lemon zest refreshes and uplifts. **Safety**: *Keep eyes closed to avoid irritation from the steam.*

Ingredients	Instructions
<ul><li>2 tbsp fresh parsley leaves</li><li>Zest of ½ lemon</li><li>3 cups hot water</li><li>Towel</li></ul>	1. Place parsley and lemon zest in a large bowl. 2. Pour hot water over them. 3. Lean over carefully with a towel over your head. 4. Inhale the steam deeply for 5–10 minutes.

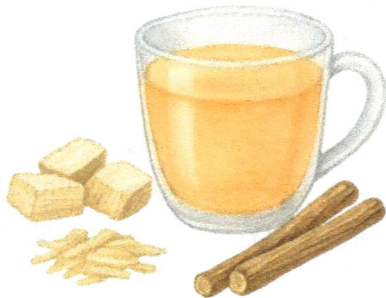

Marshmallow Root & Licorice Soothing Decoction

A soft, mucilaginous decoction that coats and calms the urinary tract. Marshmallow root eases irritation, while licorice root adds gentle sweetness and supports kidney balance.

Ingredients	Instructions
<ul><li>1 tbsp dried marshmallow root</li><li>1 tsp dried licorice root pieces</li><li>2 cups water</li></ul>	10. Place marshmallow root and licorice root in a small pot with water. 11. Bring to a gentle simmer for 15 minutes. 12. Strain and sip warm.

Headache & Migraine Soothers

A sudden headache can change the course of an entire day. You might be in the middle of answering emails when a dull pressure begins behind your temples. Or perhaps you wake up with the sharp pulse of a migraine that makes even light and sound feel unbearable. These moments make it hard to think clearly, focus on conversations, or enjoy simple activities.

Natural remedies can give you practical ways to respond. They are not meant to replace medical treatment in severe cases, but they can provide comfort when you need it most. What matters is having solutions you can prepare quickly, without complicated steps, and with ingredients you may already keep in your kitchen or bathroom cabinet.

Different situations call for different approaches:

Tension after long hours at the desk: Warm compresses or aromatic roll-ons with herbs like lavender, basil, or peppermint can relax tight muscles and ease pressure around the head and neck.

Recurring migraines that drain energy: Gentle infusions with feverfew or skullcap may offer steady support when used regularly, helping the body find more balance over time.

Headaches triggered by stress or fatigue: Soothing teas with chamomile, rose, or passionflower can calm both body and mind, reducing the emotional strain that often fuels discomfort.

Congestion-related head pressure: Steams with peppermint, rosemary, or eucalyptus open the airways and bring clarity, making it easier to breathe and think clearly again.

The remedies in this chapter are designed to fit naturally into daily life. A simple tea requires only a mug and hot water. A roll-on can be prepared once and carried in your pocket for quick use. A steam bowl can be set up in minutes when pressure builds unexpectedly. These are not elaborate treatments but straightforward tools that help you regain comfort and stability.

As you move through the recipes, choose the options that match your situation. Whether you need something calming for stress, refreshing for mental fatigue, or soothing for a sore head, the following pages will provide clear and accessible support.

Peppermint & Lavender Headache Tea

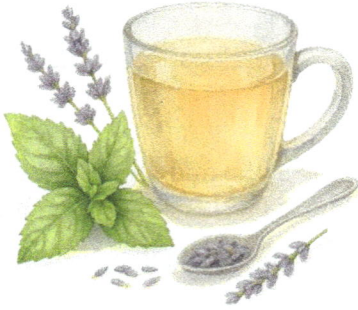

A refreshing herbal tea that cools the temples and eases tension headaches. Best enjoyed at the first signs of pressure or after a stressful day. The calming aroma can also help you shift from mental overload to a more centered state of relaxation. **Tip**: *Inhale the steam while the tea steeps for an extra calming effect.*

Ingredients	Instructions
• 1 tsp dried peppermint leaves • 1 tsp dried lavender flowers • 1 cup hot water	1. Place peppermint and lavender in a mug. 2. Pour hot water over the herbs. 3. Cover and steep for 7–8 minutes. 4. Strain and sip slowly.

Feverfew & Lemon Balm Infusion

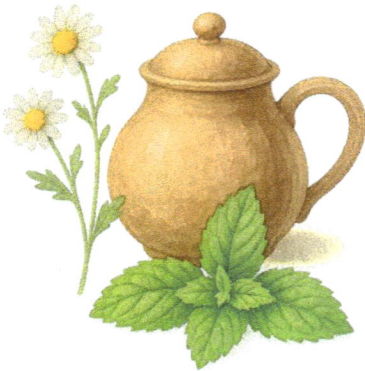

This gentle infusion provides natural support for recurring headaches. Feverfew helps soothe discomfort, while lemon balm eases nervous tension. Drinking it regularly may support long-term balance, especially for those who notice patterns in their headaches. **Safety**: *Avoid feverfew during pregnancy or if you are on blood-thinning medication.*

Ingredients	Instructions
• 1 tsp dried feverfew leaves • 1 tsp dried lemon balm leaves • 1 cup hot water	1. Combine feverfew and lemon balm in a teapot. 2. Pour hot water and cover. 3. Steep for 10 minutes, then strain

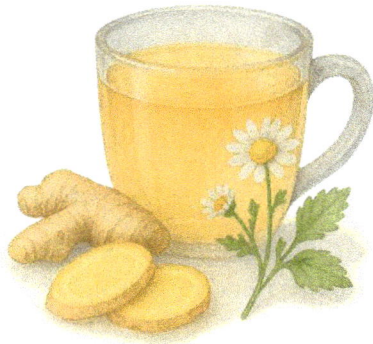

Ginger & Chamomile Comfort Tea

A warming, soothing tea that eases nausea and pressure often linked with migraines. Drink during early symptoms to calm the body and mind. The combination of spice and floral calm can also help reduce sensitivity to light and sound. **Tip**: *Drink slowly in a quiet space to maximize relief.*

Ingredients	Instructions
• 1 tsp fresh ginger slices • 1 tsp dried chamomile flowers • 1 cup hot water • 1 tsp honey (optional)	1. Place ginger and chamomile in a mug. 2. Pour hot water over them. 3. Cover and steep for 8 minutes. 4. Strain, add honey if desired, and sip warm.

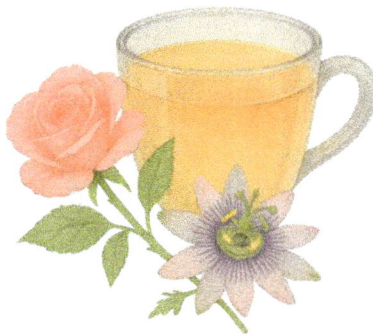

Rose & Passionflower Relaxing Brew

A fragrant blend that soothes emotional stress while calming headache tension. Rose uplifts the mood, and passionflower eases mental restlessness. This gentle brew is especially helpful when headaches are tied to worry or emotional overload. **Safety**: *Avoid passionflower if pregnant or taking sedative medications.*

Ingredients	Instructions
• 1 tsp dried rose petals • 1 tsp dried passionflower • 1 cup hot water	1. Add rose petals and passionflower to a mug. 2. Pour hot water and cover. 3. Steep for 7–8 minutes. 4. Strain and enjoy warm.

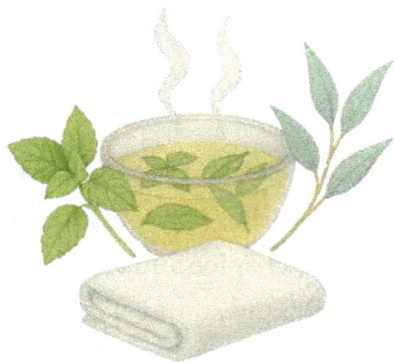

Peppermint & Eucalyptus Cooling Compress

A quick external remedy to ease forehead pressure. The cool sensation of peppermint and eucalyptus helps clear the head and reduce discomfort. It's a practical option when you cannot take time to prepare a drink but need immediate relief. **Safety**: *Avoid contact with eyes; eucalyptus may cause irritation.*

Ingredients	Instructions
<ul><li>1 tbsp dried peppermint leaves</li><li>1 tbsp dried eucalyptus leaves</li><li>2 cups hot water</li><li>1 clean cotton cloth</li></ul>	1. Place peppermint and eucalyptus in a bowl. 2. Pour hot water over the herbs and let steep for 10 minutes. 3. Strain and let cool slightly. 4. Soak the cloth, wring gently, and place on your forehead for 10–15 minutes.

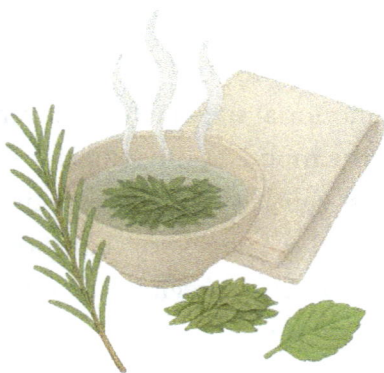

Rosemary & Peppermint Inhalation

A fresh herbal steam that awakens the mind and eases head heaviness. Rosemary stimulates clarity, while peppermint clears blocked sinuses that may trigger headaches. This method also improves circulation to the head, helping you feel lighter and more focused. **Tip**: *Keep your eyes closed to avoid irritation.*

Ingredients	Instructions
<ul><li>1 tbsp dried rosemary</li><li>1 tbsp dried peppermint leaves</li><li>3 cups hot water</li><li>Towel</li></ul>	1. Place rosemary and peppermint in a large bowl. 2. Pour hot water over them. 3. Lean over with a towel over your head. 4. Inhale the steam for 5–10 minutes.

Lavender & Basil Essential Oil Roll-On

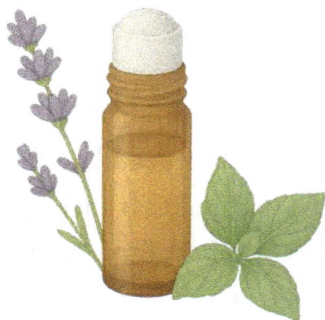

This portable roll-on calms temporal tension and eases stress. Lavender relaxes, while basil helps reduce head strain during busy days. It's small enough to keep in a pocket or bag, making it ideal for use while traveling or at work. **Safety**: *Perform a patch test before use; avoid contact with eyes.*

Ingredients	Instructions
<ul><li>10 ml roller bottle</li><li>8 drops lavender essential oil</li><li>4 drops basil essential oil</li><li>Carrier oil (such as jojoba or sweet almond)</li></ul>	1. Fill the roller bottle with carrier oil, leaving some space at the top. 2. Add lavender and basil essential oils. 3. Cap tightly and shake to blend. 4. Apply to temples, wrists, or neck as needed.

Ginger & Clove Warm Neck Compress

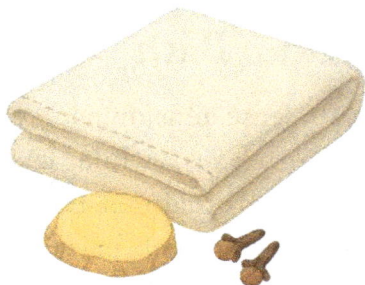

A warming compress that relaxes tense neck muscles, often a hidden trigger for headaches. Ginger increases circulation, while clove adds soothing warmth. It works especially well after long hours at the desk or when tension builds in the shoulders.

Ingredients	Instructions
<ul><li>1 tbsp fresh ginger slices</li><li>3 whole cloves</li><li>2 cups hot water</li><li>Clean cotton cloth</li></ul>	1. Place ginger and cloves in a bowl. 2. Pour hot water over them and steep for 10 minutes. 3. Strain and soak the cloth. 4. Apply warm compress to the back of the neck for 15–20 minutes.

Feverfew & Mint Herbal Capsules

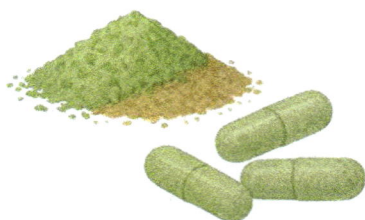

A convenient daily option for migraine support. Feverfew may help reduce frequency, while mint adds digestive comfort. Preparing capsules in advance makes it easier to stay consistent with natural support over time. **Safety**: *Do not use feverfew during pregnancy or with blood-thinning medications.*

Ingredients	Instructions
• 2 tbsp dried feverfew (powdered) • 1 tbsp dried peppermint (powdered) • Empty vegetarian capsules	1. Mix powdered feverfew and peppermint in a small bowl. 2. Fill empty capsules with the blend using a capsule machine or by hand. 3. Store in an airtight container. 4. Take 1 capsule daily with water.

Chamomile & Lemon Foot Bath

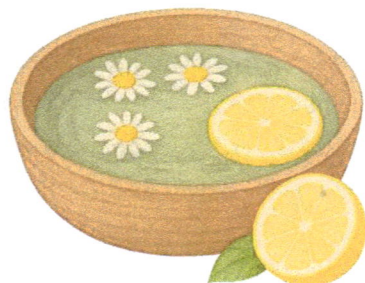

A calming foot soak that helps release tension and ease headache discomfort. Chamomile relaxes, while lemon refreshes body and mind. It's a simple ritual that not only soothes the head but also grounds the whole body before rest. **Tip**: *Use before bed to relax and support restful sleep.*

Ingredients	Instructions
• 2 tbsp dried chamomile flowers • 2 slices fresh lemon • Basin of warm water	1. Place chamomile and lemon slices in a basin. 2. Pour warm water over them. 3. Soak feet for 15–20 minutes.

Rosewater & Peppermint Eye Pad

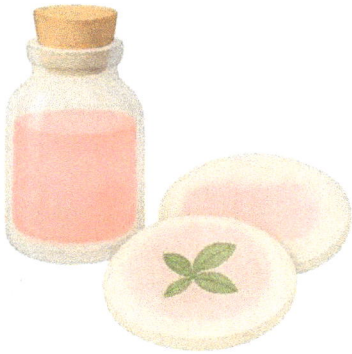

A soothing eye pad that reduces eye strain and refreshes tired eyes. Rosewater calms irritation, while peppermint cools and relieves tension. This can be especially helpful after long hours at a screen, when visual fatigue contributes to headaches. **Safety**: *Ensure oils are well diluted; avoid direct contact with eyes.*

Ingredients	Instructions
• 2 cotton pads • 2 tbsp rosewater • 2 drops peppermint essential oil (diluted in 1 tsp carrier oil)	1. Soak cotton pads in rosewater. 2. Add diluted peppermint oil to the pads. 3. Place gently over closed eyes for 10 minutes.

Willow Bark & Ginger Decoction

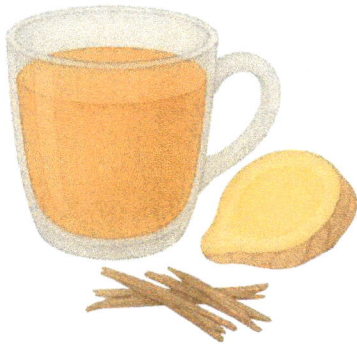

A traditional drink for natural headache relief. Willow bark provides gentle pain-soothing properties, while ginger supports circulation and comfort. Taken warm, it can ease both physical pressure and the overall heaviness of a lingering headache. **Safety**: *Avoid willow bark if allergic to aspirin or taking blood-thinning medication.*

Ingredients	Instructions
• 1 tsp dried willow bark • 1 tsp fresh ginger slices • 2 cups water	1. Place willow bark and ginger in a pot with water. 2. Simmer gently for 15 minutes. 3. Strain and sip warm.

Oral & Dental Care (Teeth & Gums)

A healthy mouth affects more than just your smile. When your teeth and gums are comfortable, eating is enjoyable, your breath feels fresh, and daily interactions flow with ease. But even small irritations can make a difference. A sore gum after flossing, a sudden toothache at night, or a dry throat after a long day of talking can all disrupt your routine.

Natural remedies offer quick, practical ways to manage these situations. You do not need complicated products filled with artificial ingredients. With herbs, spices, and a few basic tools, you can create rinses, gargles, pastes, and simple treatments that support oral comfort and hygiene.

Here are common situations where the remedies in this chapter can help:

- **After meals:** Herbal mouth rinses with sage, peppermint, or lemon peel leave your mouth feeling fresh and clean.

- **Sensitive gums:** Gentle gargles with chamomile or clove calm irritation and provide natural cleansing support.

- **Tooth discomfort:** Diluted clove oil can be applied directly for temporary relief until you reach a dentist.

- **Daily hygiene:** Homemade powders and pastes with turmeric, baking soda, or charcoal offer simple, natural ways to care for teeth.

- **On the go:** Pocket-friendly remedies like gum gels, chews, or sprays give you quick relief when brushing is not possible.

Most of these recipes take only a few minutes to prepare. A cup of hot water is enough for a mouth rinse. A small jar of honey and cloves can become a natural gargle. Even a handful of fennel seeds in your bag can freshen your breath after a meal. These are everyday solutions that work without complicating your routine.

The goal of this chapter is to give you reliable tools to support oral and dental health in simple, practical ways. Whether you want to ease mild discomfort, prevent irritation, or just feel fresher during the day, you will find clear recipes that are easy to prepare and easy to use.

Sage & Peppermint Mouth Rinse

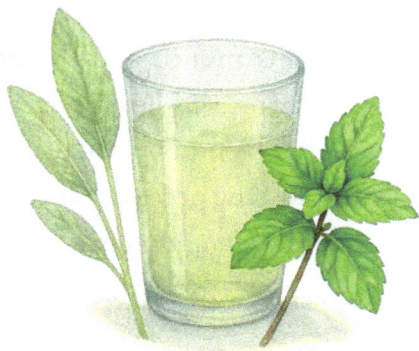

A refreshing rinse that leaves your mouth clean and invigorated. Sage purifies the gums, while peppermint delivers lasting freshness after meals. This rinse can be especially useful after consuming strong-flavored foods like garlic or coffee, helping you feel confident in social situations. **Tip**: *Use once daily after brushing for extra freshness.*

Ingredients	Instructions
• 1 tsp dried sage leaves • 1 tsp dried peppermint leaves • 1 cup hot water	1. Place sage and peppermint in a cup. 2. Pour hot water over the herbs and cover. 3. Steep for 10 minutes, then strain. 4. Allow to cool and use as a mouth rinse.

Clove & Cinnamon Antiseptic Gargle

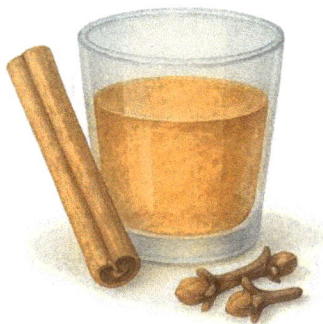

This warming gargle supports sensitive gums and freshens breath naturally. Clove brings mild numbing relief, while cinnamon adds antibacterial warmth. It can be a handy ally when you feel early signs of gum irritation or after dental cleaning. **Safety**: *Avoid swallowing the gargle; spit out after use.*

Ingredients	Instructions
• 1 small cinnamon stick • 3 whole cloves • 1 cup hot water	1. Add cloves and cinnamon stick to a cup. 2. Pour hot water over them and cover. 3. Steep for 8–10 minutes. 4. Strain, let cool slightly, and gargle for 30 seconds.

Chamomile & Saltwater Gargle

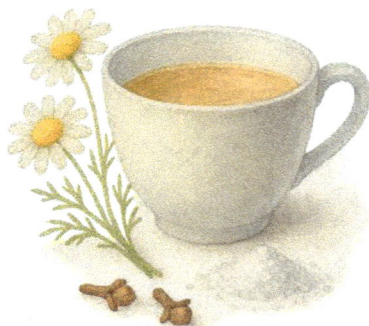

A simple yet effective gargle that calms mouth and throat irritation. Chamomile soothes discomfort, while saltwater helps cleanse and reduce swelling. This blend is particularly helpful if your gums feel tender after flossing or if your throat is scratchy from dryness. **Tip**: *Ideal after dental procedures or when gums feel sore.*

Ingredients	Instructions
<ul><li>1 tsp dried chamomile flowers</li><li>½ tsp sea salt</li><li>1 cup hot water</li></ul>	1. Brew chamomile in hot water, steep 7 minutes. 2. Strain and allow to cool. 3. Stir in salt until dissolved. 4. Gargle for 30 seconds, repeat as needed.

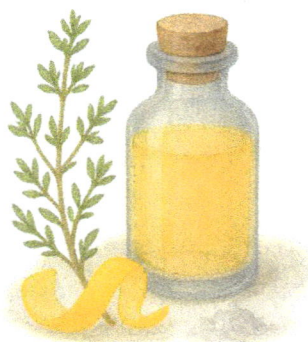

Thyme & Lemon Peel Mouthwash

This aromatic rinse supports oral hygiene while leaving a clean, citrusy aftertaste. Thyme helps cleanse the mouth, and lemon peel refreshes the breath. It's a natural alternative to conventional mouthwash, without artificial colors or alcohol. **Safety**: *Avoid use if you have known allergies to thyme.*

Ingredients	Instructions
<ul><li>1 tsp dried thyme</li><li>Zest of ½ lemon</li><li>1 cup hot water</li></ul>	1. Place thyme and lemon zest in a heat-proof jar. 2. Pour hot water over and cover. 3. Steep for 10 minutes, then strain. 4. Let cool and use as a mouthwash.

Baking Soda & Peppermint Tooth Powder

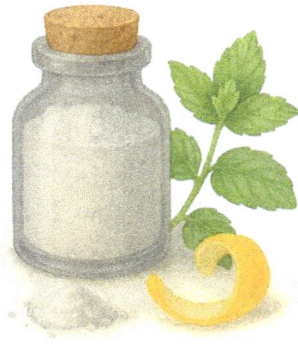

A gentle, mineral-rich powder that cleans teeth and freshens breath. Baking soda helps remove surface stains, while peppermint adds a cool, clean flavor. This powder is travel-friendly and can be a practical alternative when you don't have toothpaste at hand. **Tip**: *Use 2–3 times per week to avoid enamel abrasion.*

Ingredients	Instructions
• 2 tbsp baking soda • 1 tsp fine sea salt • 5 drops peppermint essential oil (food grade)	1. Mix baking soda and salt in a small bowl. 2. Add peppermint oil and stir well. 3. Store in a small airtight jar. 4. Dip a damp toothbrush into the powder and brush gently.

Turmeric & Coconut Oil Toothpaste

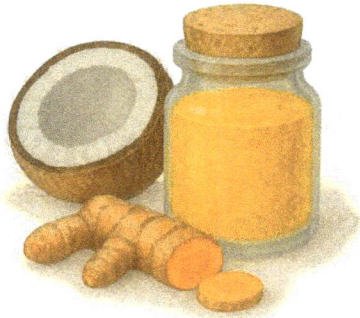

A natural paste that supports gum health while helping to reduce surface stains. Turmeric brings balance and brightness, and coconut oil keeps gums nourished. This paste can be a mild, everyday option if you want to avoid synthetic ingredients in conventional toothpaste. **Safety**: *Turmeric may temporarily stain toothbrushes or fabrics.*

Ingredients	Instructions
• 2 tbsp coconut oil (softened) • 1 tsp turmeric powder • 3 drops peppermint essential oil (optional)	1. Mix coconut oil and turmeric in a small bowl. 2. Add peppermint oil and blend until smooth. 3. Transfer to a small glass jar. 4. Use a clean spoon to apply to your toothbrush and brush gently.

Clove & Cardamom Fresh Breath Powder

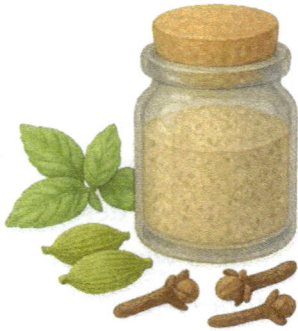

This aromatic blend helps neutralize heavy breath after meals. Clove provides a warm, spicy freshness, while cardamom seeds add a sweet, cooling lift. Keeping a jar in your bathroom allows for a quick, natural refresher when you don't want to rely on chewing gum. **Safety**: *Use sparingly to avoid gum irritation.*

Ingredients	Instructions
<ul><li>1 tsp ground clove</li><li>1 tsp ground cardamom</li><li>2 tbsp baking soda</li></ul>	1. Combine clove, cardamom, and baking soda in a small jar. 2. Mix thoroughly until even. 3. Dip a damp toothbrush into the powder. 4. Brush gently for fresh breath.

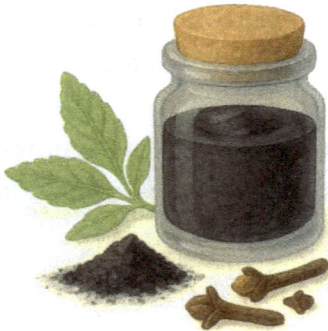

Charcoal & Sage Whitening Paste

A gentle paste that helps brighten teeth naturally. Activated charcoal binds surface stains, while sage adds a clean herbal touch for fresh breath. This blend is a chemical-free way to enhance your smile without relying on commercial whitening strips.

Ingredients	Instructions
<ul><li>1 tsp activated charcoal powder</li><li>2 tbsp coconut oil</li><li>1 tsp dried sage (powdered)</li></ul>	1. Mix coconut oil with charcoal powder. 2. Add powdered sage and stir until smooth. 3. Store in a small glass jar. 4. Apply a thin layer on your toothbrush and brush gently.

Aloe Vera & Peppermint Gum Gel

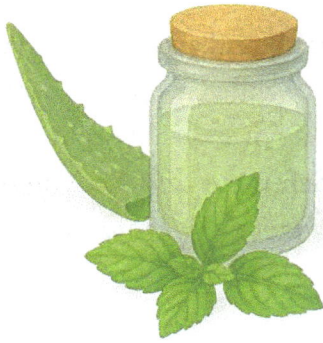

A soothing gel that calms irritated gums and refreshes the mouth. Aloe vera hydrates and comforts, while peppermint brings a cooling sensation. It's especially helpful during periods of gum sensitivity, such as after eating very hot foods. **Safety**: *Test a small area before use to avoid sensitivity.*

Ingredients	Instructions
<ul><li>2 tbsp fresh aloe vera gel</li><li>3 drops peppermint essential oil (diluted)</li></ul>	1. Place aloe gel in a small bowl. 2. Add diluted peppermint oil and stir well. 3. Store in a small glass jar. 4. Apply a pea-sized amount directly to the gums as needed.

Clove Oil Toothache Remedy

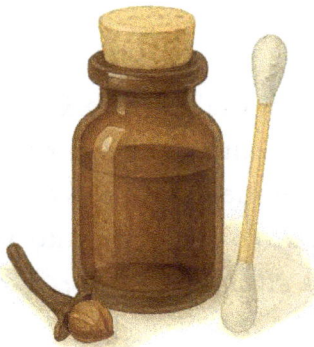

A quick natural option for localized tooth discomfort. Clove oil provides temporary numbing relief, making it useful until you can see a dentist. It works best when applied directly to the area causing pain, offering short-term comfort. **Safety**: *Never use undiluted clove oil directly on gums; it may cause irritation.*

Ingredients	Instructions
<ul><li>2 drops clove essential oil</li><li>1 tsp carrier oil (such as olive or coconut)</li><li>Cotton ball or swab</li></ul>	1. Mix clove oil with carrier oil. 2. Soak a cotton ball or swab in the blend. 3. Apply gently to the affected tooth or gum for a few minutes.

Myrrh & Calendula Gum Rinse

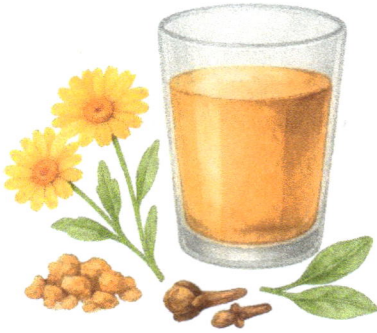

This gentle rinse supports gum health and calms sensitivity. Myrrh tones and protects the gums, while calendula soothes and promotes comfort. It can be part of a weekly routine to maintain strong, resilient gums. **Safety**: *Avoid swallowing; not recommended during pregnancy without medical guidance.*

Ingredients	Instructions
<ul><li>1 tsp myrrh resin (powdered or tincture)</li><li>1 tsp dried calendula petals</li><li>1 cup hot water</li></ul>	1. Place calendula in a cup and pour hot water over it. 2. Steep for 10 minutes, then strain. 3. Add a few drops of myrrh tincture or a pinch of powdered resin. 4. Swish as a mouth rinse and spit out.

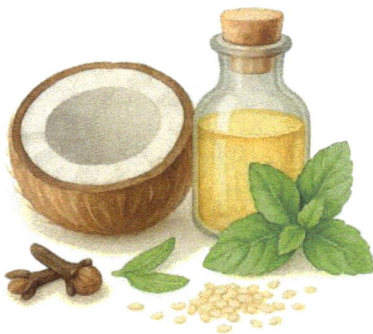

Coconut Oil Pulling Blend (Sesame & Mint)

An ancient practice that supports daily oral hygiene. Coconut and sesame oils help cleanse the mouth, while mint adds freshness. This simple habit can be done while showering or preparing breakfast, making it easy to integrate into your morning routine. **Safety**: *Do not swallow the oil; discard properly to avoid clogging drains.*

Ingredients	Instructions
<ul><li>1 tbsp coconut oil</li><li>1 tsp sesame oil</li><li>2 drops peppermint essential oil (optional, food grade)</li></ul>	1. Combine coconut oil and sesame oil in a small jar. 2. Add peppermint oil if desired and stir well. 3. Place 1 tbsp in your mouth and swish for 5–10 minutes. 4. Spit out into a tissue or bin (not the sink).

Natural First Aid Kit

S mall accidents are part of everyday life. A scraped knee while gardening, an insect bite during a walk, or a splash of hot liquid in the kitchen can appear without warning. In those moments, what helps most is having something ready at hand, simple to use, and quick to apply.

A natural first aid kit offers exactly that. By preparing a few remedies in advance, you can respond right away instead of waiting or improvising. The ingredients are familiar and easy to store: honey, aloe, chamomile, lavender, salt, vinegar, or a handful of seeds. With these basics, you can create small but effective solutions that bring comfort when you need it most.

The recipes in this chapter are organized to cover the most common situations you may face at home or while traveling:

- **Cuts and scrapes:** Creams and salves with calendula or comfrey that help soothe and protect the skin.

- **Burns and sun exposure:** Cooling gels and oils with aloe, cucumber, or St. John's wort that ease heat and calm irritation.

- **Insect bites and rashes:** Simple poultices and sprays with plantain, basil, or tea tree to reduce itching and discomfort.

- **Sudden upsets:** Quick teas, chews, or inhalers with ginger, fennel, or peppermint for mild nausea, indigestion, or headaches.

- **Eye and sinus comfort:** Gentle washes and steams with rosewater, thyme, or eucalyptus that refresh and restore ease.

Each preparation is designed with practicality in mind. A tin of salve can be kept in your bag, a spray can stay in your car, and a small jar of seeds can sit in your kitchen drawer. This way, you are not only ready for unexpected moments but also able to handle them calmly and effectively.

The following pages will guide you through fast, reliable remedies to build your own natural first aid kit. With just a little preparation, you can create a personal set of supports that makes daily life easier and gives you peace of mind.

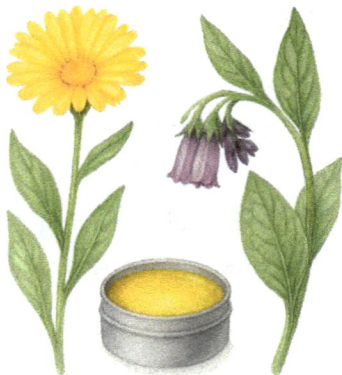

Calendula & Comfrey Healing Salve

A nourishing salve that supports skin repair after small cuts or scrapes. Calendula calms redness and discomfort, while comfrey helps the skin knit back together naturally. Keeping a small tin ready means you can address minor injuries right away instead of letting them worsen. **Safety**: *Do not use comfrey on deep or infected wounds.*

Ingredients	Instructions
<ul><li>2 tbsp calendula-infused oil</li><li>2 tbsp comfrey-infused oil</li><li>1 tbsp beeswax</li></ul>	1. Melt beeswax gently in a double boiler. 2. Stir in calendula and comfrey oils until smooth. 3. Pour into a small tin and let solidify. 4. Apply a thin layer to clean, minor cuts as needed.

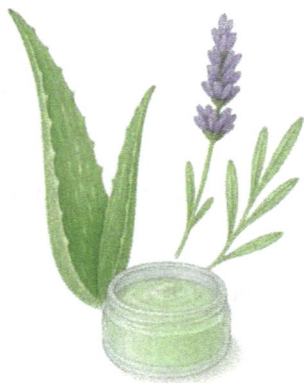

Aloe Vera & Lavender Soothing Gel

A cooling gel that eases irritation and hydrates freshly scraped skin. Aloe offers gentle moisture, while lavender's calming scent helps reduce stress at the same time. Having this gel on hand is practical for summer outings when small accidents and sun exposure are common. **Tip**: *Keep refrigerated for an extra cooling effect.*

Ingredients	Instructions
<ul><li>2 tbsp fresh aloe vera gel</li><li>3 drops lavender essential oil (diluted)</li></ul>	1. Place aloe vera gel in a clean bowl. 2. Add diluted lavender oil and stir well. 3. Store in a small jar and apply directly to the affected area.

Honey & Turmeric Antiseptic Paste

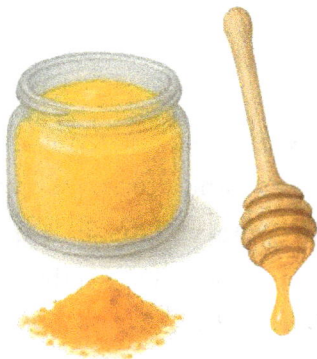

This golden paste protects minor wounds with a natural antimicrobial shield. Honey soothes the skin, while turmeric supports recovery with its warming, balancing qualities. It's a quick solution when you need to cover a scrape and don't have commercial ointment nearby. **Safety**: *Turmeric may stain skin and fabrics; use sparingly.*

Ingredients	Instructions
• 1 tsp raw honey • ½ tsp turmeric powder	1. Mix honey and turmeric in a small bowl to form a thick paste. 2. Apply a thin layer to the cut after cleaning. 3. Cover lightly with a clean bandage if needed.

Aloe & Peppermint Cooling Gel

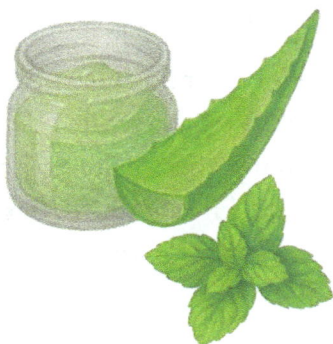

This refreshing gel offers instant relief after a minor burn or sunburn. Aloe helps the skin retain moisture, while peppermint provides a cooling sensation that reduces discomfort. It's especially useful to keep in the fridge so you're ready for hot summer days. **Safety**: *Use only on minor burns; avoid open or severe wounds.*

Ingredients	Instructions
• 2 tbsp fresh aloe vera gel • 2 drops peppermint essential oil (diluted)	1. Place aloe vera gel in a bowl. 2. Add diluted peppermint oil and stir well. 3. Apply gently over the affected skin.

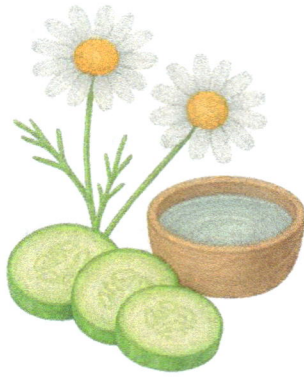

Chamomile & Cucumber Compress

A soothing compress that calms overheated or sun-exposed skin. Chamomile reduces redness and tension, while cucumber hydrates and cools on contact. This is a quick, natural option after spending time outdoors, especially when shade and water aren't enough. **Tip**: *Chill the infusion before use for a stronger cooling effect.*

Ingredients	Instructions
• 2 tbsp dried chamomile flowers (or 2 tea bags) • ½ cucumber, sliced • 1 cup cool water • Clean cotton cloth	1. Brew chamomile tea and let it cool completely. 2. Place cucumber slices into the cooled liquid. 3. Soak the cloth, wring out excess, and apply to the skin for 10–15 minutes.

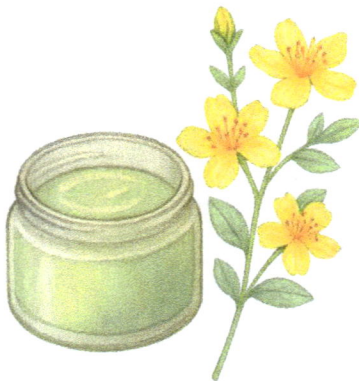

St. John's Wort Oil Burn Relief

A calming oil blend that brings relief to mild burns or sun irritation. St. John's wort supports skin repair, while olive oil locks in moisture and protects. Having this ready at home means you can act quickly after a small kitchen burn. **Safety**: *Do not use on severe burns; seek medical help for serious injuries.*

Ingredients	Instructions
• 2 tbsp St. John's wort–infused oil • 1 tsp aloe vera gel	1. Combine St. John's wort oil and aloe gel in a small bowl. 2. Stir until smooth. 3. Apply gently to minor burns once the skin has cooled with water.

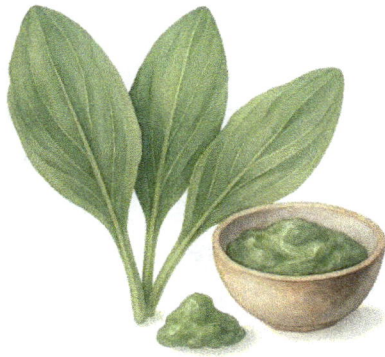

Plantain Leaf Poultice

A quick herbal paste that eases itching and swelling from insect bites or minor skin irritations. Plantain leaves release a soothing juice that can calm the skin almost instantly. It's an easy solution when you're outdoors and need relief on the spot. **Tip**: *If fresh leaves are available, chewing them lightly before applying can help release more of their soothing juices.*

Ingredients	Instructions
• 2–3 fresh plantain leaves • A small amount of clean water	1. Crush the fresh leaves into a moist paste with clean hands or a mortar and pestle. 2. Apply directly to the bite or irritated area. 3. Hold in place for 10–15 minutes, then rinse.

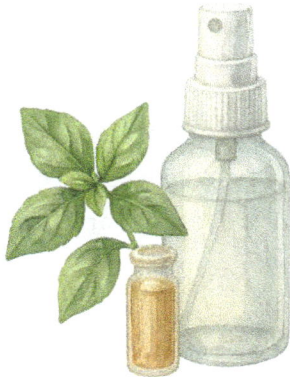

Basil & Vinegar Itch Relief Spray

This simple spray refreshes and calms itchy bites or rashes. Basil's natural oils ease irritation, while vinegar offers a cleansing and cooling effect. It's convenient for travel or camping since it can be made quickly with kitchen staples. **Safety**: *Avoid spraying on broken or very sensitive skin.*

Ingredients	Instructions
• ½ cup distilled water • 1 tbsp apple cider vinegar • 1 tbsp fresh basil leaves (lightly crushed)	1. Place basil leaves in a small jar and cover with vinegar. Let infuse for 1 hour, then strain. 2. Mix the infused vinegar with distilled water in a spray bottle. 3. Shake well before use and spritz lightly on the affected area.

Tea Tree & Lavender Roll-On

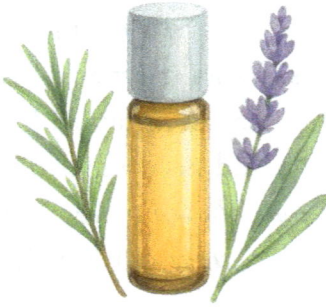

A handy roll-on that combines cleansing and soothing benefits. Tea tree helps keep small bites or scratches clean, while lavender reduces discomfort and adds a calming scent. It's pocket-sized, making it easy to carry during hikes or trips. **Safety**: *Always patch-test essential oils before use; avoid eyes and mouth.*

Ingredients	Instructions
• 10 ml roller bottle • 5 drops tea tree essential oil • 5 drops lavender essential oil • Carrier oil (such as sweet almond)	1. Fill the roller bottle with carrier oil. 2. Add essential oils and shake gently. 3. Apply directly to itchy or irritated spots as needed.

Ginger & Mint Nausea Tea

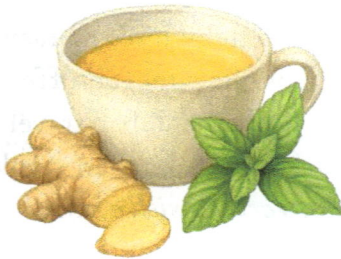

A warming yet refreshing tea that settles the stomach during travel or mild nausea. Ginger supports smoother digestion, while mint eases queasiness. Keeping dried slices in your bag makes it easy to brew a quick cup wherever you are. **Tip**: *Sip in small amounts to calm your stomach gently.*

Ingredients	Instructions
• 1 tsp fresh grated ginger • 1 tsp fresh mint leaves • 1 cup hot water	1. Place ginger and mint in a cup. 2. Pour hot water over the herbs and cover. 3. Steep for 7–8 minutes, then strain and sip slowly.

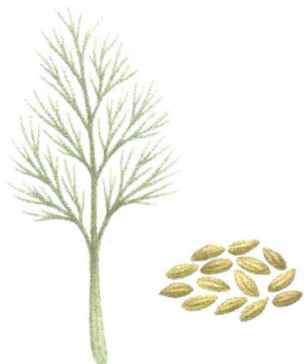

Fennel Seed Chew for Indigestion

A fast and traditional remedy for post-meal heaviness. Chewing fennel seeds can relieve gas, support digestion, and leave your breath pleasantly fresh. Keep a small tin of seeds in your bag or car for easy access after eating. **Safety**: *Avoid excess fennel if pregnant without medical advice.*

Ingredients	Instructions
1 tsp fennel seeds (lightly toasted if desired)	1. Take a small spoonful of fennel seeds. 2. Chew slowly after meals. 3. Swallow or discard the fibers as preferred.

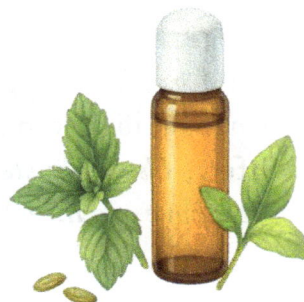

Peppermint & Lemon Balm Headache Inhaler

A portable inhaler that helps ease mild headaches and tension. Peppermint's cooling effect clears the head, while lemon balm relaxes the body and calms the mind. It's especially useful when you're on the go and need quick relief without medication. **Safety**: *Not suitable for children under 6; avoid contact with eyes.*

Ingredients	Instructions
• 5 drops peppermint essential oil • 5 drops lemon balm essential oil • 1 cotton wick or pad • 1 small inhaler tube	1. Insert cotton wick into the inhaler tube. 2. Add essential oils to the wick. 3. Inhale gently whenever a mild headache arises.

Clove Oil Toothache Remedy

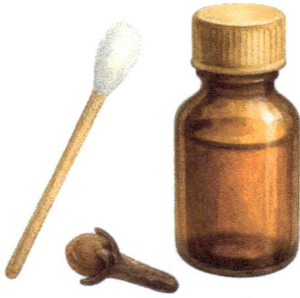

A quick, natural option to calm sudden tooth pain before you can see a dentist. Clove oil provides temporary numbing relief, making it easier to manage discomfort. Having a pre-mixed bottle ensures you're ready if toothache strikes at night. **Safety**: *Never apply undiluted clove oil directly on gums.*

Ingredients	Instructions
• 2 drops clove essential oil • 1 tsp carrier oil (such as olive or coconut) • Cotton ball or swab	1. Mix clove oil with carrier oil. 2. Soak the cotton ball or swab in the blend. 3. Apply gently to the affected tooth or gum for a few minutes.

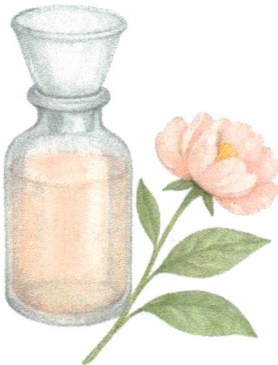

Rosewater Eye Wash

A gentle rinse that refreshes tired or irritated eyes. Rosewater soothes redness and provides cooling comfort after a long day of screen use or exposure to wind. Using it at night can help your eyes feel rested before sleep. **Safety**: *Use only sterile, preservative-free rosewater; avoid if you have eye infections or injuries.*

Ingredients	Instructions
• ½ cup pure rosewater (sterile, preservative-free) • Sterile eye cup or dropper	1. Pour rosewater into a sterile eye cup or use a clean dropper. 2. Gently rinse the eye by tilting your head back and blinking a few times. 3. Discard any unused liquid after each use.

Eucalyptus & Thyme Steam

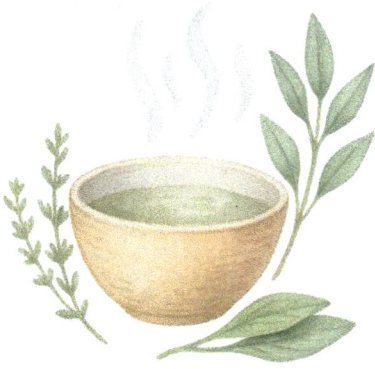

A fast-acting steam that helps open congested sinuses and ease sudden breathing discomfort. Eucalyptus clears the airways, while thyme brings a refreshing herbal lift. This quick remedy can be prepared in minutes with simple kitchen tools. **Safety**: *Keep eyes closed while inhaling steam; not suitable for young children.*

Ingredients	Instructions
• 1 tbsp dried thyme • 1 tbsp dried eucalyptus leaves • 3 cups hot water • Towel	1. Place thyme and eucalyptus in a large bowl. 2. Pour hot water over them. 3. Lean over with a towel over your head and inhale deeply for 5–10 minutes.

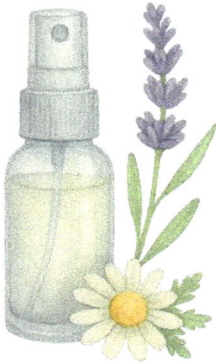

Lavender & Chamomile Hand Soothe Mist

A light mist that refreshes and comforts hands after frequent washing or contact with cleaning products. Lavender calms irritation, while chamomile eases dryness and supports soft, supple skin. It's a practical remedy to carry in your bag for quick relief throughout the day. **Tip**: *Store in the fridge for a cooling effect, especially in summer.*

Ingredients	Instructions
• ½ cup distilled water • 1 tbsp chamomile tea (strongly brewed and cooled) • 5 drops lavender essential oil • 1 small spray bottle	1. Brew chamomile tea and let it cool completely. 2. Pour the tea into a clean spray bottle with distilled water. 3. Add lavender essential oil and shake gently. 4. Spray lightly on your hands and let air-dry.

Part 3 – Integrating Natural Healing

H aving a collection of remedies is valuable, but the real benefits appear when you make them part of your everyday rhythm. Natural healing is not about one-time solutions, it is about steady habits that keep your body balanced and your mind clear over time. This section will show you how to move from trying recipes occasionally to living with them in a consistent, sustainable way.

Daily routines often leave little space for self-care, which is why structure matters. A morning drink, a calming evening tea, or a weekly bath can become anchors in your schedule, guiding your body toward balance without requiring extra effort. By repeating these small actions, you create signals your body begins to recognize, making relaxation, focus, and renewal more natural.

Here are some ways this section will help you put remedies into practice:

- **Morning routines:** Start the day with a simple drink that supports energy and clarity, or use a refreshing spray before work.

- **Evening practices:** Choose calming infusions or relaxing baths that signal your body it is time to rest.

- **Weekly care:** Set aside moments for deeper support, such as a mineral-rich broth or a nourishing oil treatment for skin or hair.

- **Tracking progress:** Learn how to keep a simple journal to notice changes in mood, energy, or comfort over time.

The recipes here are meant to be flexible. You can try them one at a time, see how your body responds, and then decide which ones fit naturally into your lifestyle. Some people find that a single evening tea improves their sleep, while others benefit from combining a morning tonic with a weekly soak. What matters is not doing everything, but creating a routine that works for you.

This part of the book is about connection. It connects the knowledge you have gained in the first section with the practical recipes you explored in the second. Most importantly, it connects those remedies with your real life, so they become tools you use regularly rather than ideas you only read about.

The following chapters will give you clear suggestions for daily, weekly, and seasonal practices. They are simple, adaptable, and designed to fit into the flow of your days. By weaving them into your routine, you turn natural healing from occasional relief into a steady foundation for lasting well-being.

Daily & Weekly Healing Routines

You've now collected more than two hundred natural remedies. The next step is learning how to bring them into your daily rhythm so they don't just stay on the page. This chapter offers ready-made examples of morning, evening, and weekly routines that show how these remedies can work together.

These are not fixed schedules but practical models. Use them as a reference, then adapt them to your own lifestyle, season, and needs. The point is to see how simple it is to combine a drink, a spray, or a bath into short rituals that support balance throughout the day.

Morning Routine

Morning Lemon & Ginger Warm Water

A simple ritual to wake up the body, flush overnight stagnation, and gently kickstart metabolism. Drink it before breakfast, on an empty stomach.

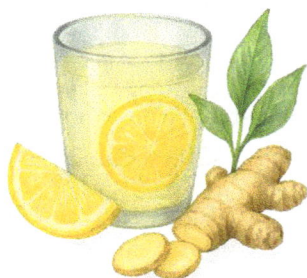

Ingredients	Instructions
1 cup warm water	Warm the water to a comfortable drinking temperature.
1 slice fresh lemon	Add lemon to the water.
2–3 slices fresh ginger	Drop in the ginger, let sit for 2–3 minutes, then sip slowly.

Mint & Rosemary Focus Spray

Use this aromatic spray right after your shower or just before starting work. It sharpens attention and creates a clear mental space to begin the day.

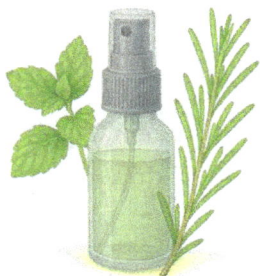

Ingredients	Instructions
½ cup distilled water	Pour water into a clean spray bottle.
5 drops peppermint essential oil	Add peppermint oil.
3 drops rosemary essential oil	Add rosemary oil, shake well before each use.

Evening Routine

Chamomile & Oat Evening Tea

This calming blend eases tension and signals your body that it's time to slow down. Best enjoyed 30–40 minutes before bed.

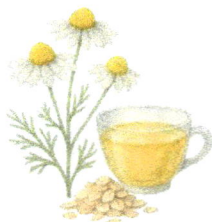

Ingredients	Instructions
1 tsp dried chamomile flowers	Place in a mug.
1 tsp rolled oats	Add oats to the mug.
1 cup hot water	Pour hot water, cover, steep 7–8 minutes. Strain and sip warm.

Lavender & Epsom Salt Foot Soak

A short but deeply relaxing evening ritual. It calms the nervous system, softens the muscles, and prepares the body for rest.

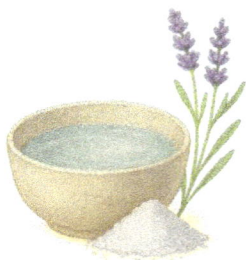

Ingredients	Instructions
1 basin warm water	Fill a basin to ankle level.
1 cup Epsom salt	Dissolve in the warm water.
2 tbsp dried lavender flowers	Add lavender, let steep a few minutes before soaking feet 15–20 minutes.

Weekly Routine

Cucumber & Aloe Hydrating Face Mask

A once-a-week ritual that restores hydration and freshness to your skin. Ideal for Sundays or a self-care evening.

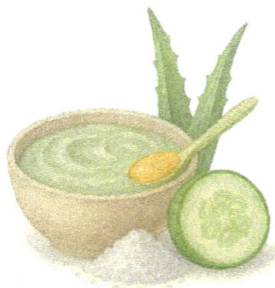

Ingredients	Instructions
½ cucumber, blended	Blend until smooth.
2 tbsp fresh aloe vera gel	Mix with cucumber pulp.
1 tsp honey (optional)	Stir in for extra nourishment. Apply to clean skin, leave for 10–15 minutes, rinse with lukewarm water.

Turmeric & Honey Weekly Detox Shot

A concentrated shot that supports natural balance and resilience. Best taken once or twice per week, preferably in the morning.

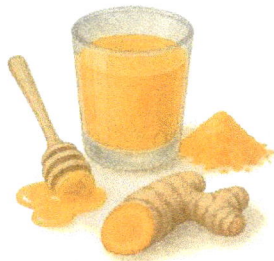

Ingredients	Instructions
½ cup warm water	Pour into a small glass.
½ tsp turmeric powder	Stir until dissolved.
1 tsp raw honey	Blend in honey, drink immediately.

How to Use These Routines

The routines in this chapter are examples, designed to show how remedies can work together in real life. Use them as inspiration, then adjust to fit your own needs. Here are some simple guidelines to help you build routines that last:

- **Anchor your mornings with one energizing ritual**: choose a drink that wakes the body, or a spray that clears the mind. If you have time, do both; if not, pick the one that matters most to you.

- **Close your evenings with calm**: combine a soothing tea with a foot soak, or alternate them depending on your schedule. The goal is to send your body a clear signal that the day is done.

- **Schedule a weekly reset**: a detox drink, a nourishing broth, or a skin mask once or twice a week keeps your system refreshed and gives you a sense of renewal.

- **Adapt to your context**: busy week? Keep it minimal. Quieter weekend? Add an extra ritual. Adjusting prevents routines from becoming a burden.

- **Stay seasonal**: lighter infusions in summer, warming broths in winter, refreshing sprays in spring. Matching remedies to the season keeps them enjoyable.

What matters most is consistency and personal fit. Start with small steps, notice which practices make you feel better, and let those become your anchors. Over time, you'll have a set of routines that are entirely yours — shaped by your needs, supported by nature, and simple enough to repeat.

Building Your Herbal Lifestyle

You've seen how remedies can be used day by day. Now the question is: how do you make them part of your life long term? Lasting benefits come not from a single tea or compress, but from the quiet rhythm of habits you actually keep. This chapter gives you tools to start small, stay consistent, and adapt along the way, so natural healing becomes part of your lifestyle rather than an occasional choice.

The simplest way to succeed is to begin with one or two remedies you enjoy. A daily cup of tea before bed. A refreshing infusion in the morning. A nourishing broth once a week. Choose one anchor and repeat it until it feels automatic.

Consistency matters more than variety at the beginning. Even a single practice, repeated daily, can have a cumulative effect on mood, energy, and resilience. Once that's steady, add another ritual. Think of it as layering — one practice at a time until you've built a routine that suits your rhythm.

Tracking how remedies affect you makes the experience more personal and effective. Keep a simple notebook or a page in your phone where you jot down what you tried and how you felt afterward.

Example:

Date	Remedy	How I Felt	Notes
March 3	Chamomile tea	Slept more deeply	Felt calmer in the morning
March 5	Ginger shot	Warmth, more energy	Mild stomach comfort

Herbal Journal

Date	Remedy	How I Felt	Notes

Date	Remedy	How I Felt	Notes

Seasonal Adjustments

Your body responds differently across the year, and your remedies should shift too. In summer, cooling infusions with cucumber, mint, or hibiscus help with hydration. In winter, warming drinks with ginger, cinnamon, or turmeric provide comfort and circulation. Spring invites cleansing teas with nettle or dandelion; autumn benefits from immune-supportive blends with elderberry or garlic.

You don't have to reinvent your whole routine each season. Simply swap one element: change your evening tea, adjust your weekly broth, or rotate the herbs in your infusions. The index of this book is your guide, return to it when the season changes and pick remedies that match the climate and your needs.

Building Your Herbal First-Aid Corner

Every home benefits from a small, permanent herbal first-aid kit. By now, you know how a salve, a soothing gel, or a simple tea can bring quick relief. Having them ready means you don't wait until discomfort strikes to prepare something.

Set aside a shelf or a box for:

- A few jars of dried herbs you use most often.
- Small bottles for oils, tinctures, or sprays.
- Labels with dates so you always know what's fresh.
- A simple rotation: remake small batches every few months instead of storing large quantities.

This small corner in your home becomes a source of reassurance. You'll know that comfort is within reach, with safe and familiar remedies that are already part of your lifestyle.

BONUS: Extra Lifestyle Recipes

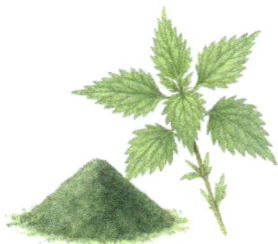

Daily Green Mineral Blend (Nettle & Spirulina Powder)

A mineral-rich mix that boosts smoothies or juices with daily nourishment. It delivers gentle energy and steady mineral support, especially useful if your diet feels low in greens.

Ingredients	Instructions
• 1 tbsp dried nettle powder • 1 tsp spirulina powder	1. Combine nettle and spirulina in a clean glass jar. 2. Store in a cool, dark place. 3. Stir 1 teaspoon of the blend into a smoothie or fresh juice once a day.

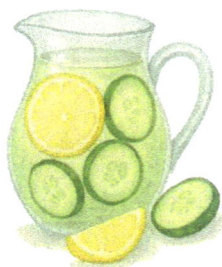

Morning Detox Water (Lemon & Cucumber Infusion)

A refreshing daily drink that supports hydration and gentle cleansing. It's light enough to sip throughout the morning, keeping your body awake without stimulants.

Ingredients	Instructions
• ½ cucumber, sliced • 2 slices fresh lemon • 1 liter cold water	1. Place cucumber and lemon slices in a large jug. 2. Cover with water and let infuse for 20 minutes. 3. Keep chilled and drink slowly during the morning.

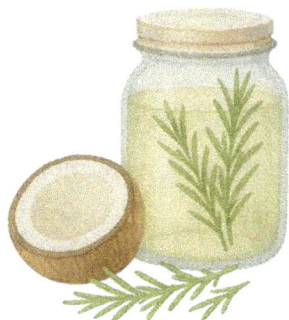

Weekly Herbal Hair Oil (Coconut & Rosemary)

A nourishing oil that strengthens hair and scalp. Use once a week to support growth, reduce dryness, and give hair a natural shine. **Note**: *Regular scalp massage also stimulates circulation, making this practice beneficial beyond the oil itself.*

Ingredients	Instructions
• ½ cup coconut oil (lightly warmed) • 2 tbsp dried rosemary	1. Place rosemary in a small jar and cover with warm coconut oil. 2. Seal and let infuse for two weeks, then strain into a clean bottle. 3. Massage a small amount into the scalp once a week, leave for 30 minutes, then rinse with mild shampoo.

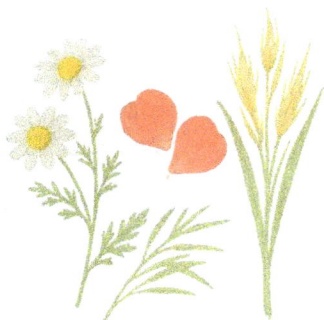

Bedtime Ritual Tea (Chamomile, Rose & Oatstraw)

A gentle nightly tea that signals your body to relax. It combines chamomile's calm, rose's soothing fragrance, and oatstraw's mineral support for deeper rest. **Note**: *Keeping this blend pre-mixed in a jar saves time and turns your evening tea into a nightly ritual instead of an occasional treat.*

Ingredients	Instructions
• 1 tsp dried chamomile flowers • 1 tsp dried rose petals • 1 tbsp dried oatstraw • 1 cup hot water	1. Place the chamomile, rose, and oatstraw in a mug. 2. Pour hot water over the herbs, cover, and steep for 7–8 minutes. 3. Strain and drink about 30 minutes before bed.

Immunity Support Soup (Garlic, Ginger & Vegetables)

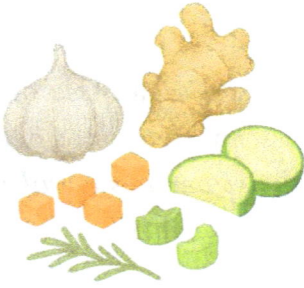

A weekly dish that nourishes while reinforcing resilience. It provides warmth, minerals, and comfort, making it a simple way to support your system through colder seasons.

Ingredients	Instructions
• 2 garlic cloves, minced • 1 tsp fresh grated ginger • 2 cups chopped seasonal vegetables (carrots, celery, zucchini, or similar) • 4 cups water or broth	1. Heat a pot and sauté garlic and ginger for 1–2 minutes. 2. Add vegetables and water or broth. 3. Simmer gently for 20 minutes, season lightly, and enjoy warm.

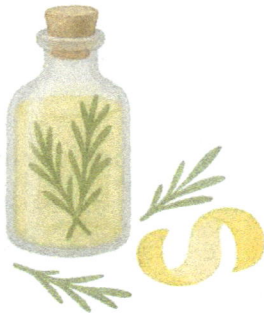

Seasonal Herbal Vinegar (Rosemary & Lemon Peel)

A simple condiment with digestive benefits. Adding it to salads or vegetables makes every meal a small act of support for your body. **Note:** *Because it keeps for months, this vinegar is a practical way to weave herbs into your diet daily without extra preparation.*

Ingredients	Instructions
• 1 cup apple cider vinegar • 2 sprigs fresh rosemary • Peel of 1 lemon	1. Place rosemary and lemon peel in a clean glass jar. 2. Cover completely with apple cider vinegar. 3. Seal, let infuse for two weeks, then strain and store. 4. Use as a dressing or drizzle over cooked vegetables.

A Final Word

"Small acts, when multiplied by millions of people, can transform the world." - Howard Zinn

When you share your thoughts about what you've read, you're not only supporting the author, you're extending a hand to someone who may be standing exactly where you once stood: searching for clarity, comfort, or a healthier rhythm.

Most people decide whether to open a book based on reviews. That means your voice can become the reason another reader finds the tools they need to sleep better, manage stress, or feel more balanced.

Would you help in that way? It won't cost you anything, and it takes less than a minute. Yet the impact could be enormous:

- One more person discovering natural support for everyday challenges.

- One more life touched by a simple, honest recommendation.

- One more step toward building a community of readers who share knowledge and care.

I appreciate every review, whether positive or critical, and I read each one personally. Your words will help others decide if this is right for them — and that alone can make a difference.

Thank you for considering it.

Scan to leave a review

References & Resources

- Ackermann, R. T., & Mulrow, C. D. (2002). Herbal medicines for sleep disorders. *Annals of Internal Medicine, 136*(1), 42–53.
- Aggarwal, B. B., & Harikumar, K. B. (2009). Potential therapeutic effects of curcumin, the anti-inflammatory agent from turmeric. *International Journal of Biochemistry & Cell Biology, 41*(1), 40–59.
- Akram, M., et al. (2018). Antiviral potential of medicinal plants against human viruses. *Journal of Clinical Medicine, 7*(3), 94.
- American Botanical Council. (2013). *Herbal medicine: Expanded Commission E monographs*. Integrative Medicine Communications.
- Bent, S., & Ko, R. (2004). Commonly used herbal medicines in the United States: A review. *American Journal of Medicine, 116*(7), 478–485.
- Blumenthal, M., et al. (2000). *Herbal Medicine: Expanded Commission E Monographs*. Integrative Medicine Communications.
- Bone, K., & Mills, S. (2013). *Principles and practice of phytotherapy* (2nd ed.). Churchill Livingstone.
- Bruneton, J. (1999). *Pharmacognosy, phytochemistry, medicinal plants* (2nd ed.). Lavoisier.
- Chevallier, A. (2016). *Encyclopedia of herbal medicine* (3rd ed.). DK Publishing.
- Cochrane Database of Systematic Reviews. (2019). Herbal interventions for insomnia. *Cochrane Library*.
- Committee on Herbal Medicinal Products (HMPC). (2016). *Assessment reports on medicinal plants*. European Medicines Agency.
- Dang, H., et al. (2007). Neuroprotective and stress-relieving properties of ginseng. *Journal of Ethnopharmacology, 111*(3), 495–502.
- Dharmananda, S. (2002). *Chinese herbs in the western clinic*. Institute for Traditional Medicine.
- Duke, J. (2002). *Handbook of medicinal herbs* (2nd ed.). CRC Press.
- Ernst, E. (2002). Herbal medicines: Balancing benefits and risks. *Novartis Foundation Symposium, 282*, 154–167.
- Foster, S., & Duke, J. (2014). *A field guide to medicinal plants and herbs of North America* (2nd ed.). Houghton Mifflin.
- Garg, A., & Gupta, D. (2015). Licorice root and its therapeutic uses. *International Journal of Herbal Medicine, 3*(2), 123–126.
- Gaster, B., & Holroyd, J. (2000). St. John's wort for depression: A systematic review. *Archives of Internal Medicine, 160*(2), 152–156.
- Goetz, C. M. (2019). Adaptogens and stress modulation. *Journal of Herbal Pharmacotherapy, 19*(4), 331–342.
- Gruenwald, J., Brendler, T., & Jaenicke, C. (2004). *PDR for herbal medicines* (4th ed.). Thomson.
- Halberstein, R. A. (2005). Medicinal plants: Historical and cross-cultural usage patterns. *Annual Review of Anthropology, 34*(1), 173–194.
- Hoffmann, D. (2003). *Medical herbalism: The science and practice of herbal medicine*. Healing Arts Press.
- Hudson, T. (2009). Botanicals and women's health. *Integrative Medicine, 8*(2), 34–42.
- Jiang, W. Y. (2005). Therapeutic wisdom in traditional Chinese medicine. *Phytotherapy Research, 19*(9), 819–823.
- Kennedy, D. O., et al. (2001). The anxiolytic effects of valerian. *Pharmacology Biochemistry and Behavior, 69*(3–4), 399–410.
- Kumar, V., & Khanum, F. (2012). Medicinal plants for digestive health. *Journal of Ayurveda and Integrative Medicine, 3*(3), 144–152.
- Langhorst, J., et al. (2013). Ginger in the treatment of irritable bowel syndrome. *Alimentary Pharmacology & Therapeutics, 37*(5), 490–500.
- Linde, K., et al. (2005). Echinacea for preventing and treating the common cold. *Cochrane Database of Systematic Reviews*.
- McIntyre, A. (2005). *Herbal treatment of children: Western and Ayurvedic perspectives*. Elsevier.
- Mills, S., & Bone, K. (2000). *The essential guide to herbal safety*. Churchill Livingstone.
- Murray, M. T., & Pizzorno, J. (2012). *Textbook of natural medicine* (4th ed.). Churchill Livingstone.
- National Center for Complementary and Integrative Health (NCCIH). (2020). *Herbs at a glance*. NIH.
- Newall, C. A., Anderson, L. A., & Phillipson, J. D. (1996). *Herbal medicines: A guide for healthcare professionals*. Pharmaceutical Press.
- Panossian, A., & Wikman, G. (2010). Effects of adaptogens on the central nervous system and fatigue. *Current Clinical Pharmacology, 5*(3), 198–219.
- Perry, N., & Perry, E. (2006). Aromatherapy in the management of psychiatric disorders. *CNS Drugs, 20*(4), 257–280.
- Romm, A. (2017). *Botanical medicine for women's health* (2nd ed.). Elsevier.
- Romm, A. (2010). *Naturally healthy babies and children*. Ten Speed Press.
- Ross, S. M. (2010). Adaptogens: A review of their history and clinical application. *Alternative Medicine Review, 15*(3), 240–251.
- Sarris, J., et al. (2011). Herbal medicines for psychiatric disorders: A systematic review. *Australian & New Zealand Journal of Psychiatry, 45*(11), 993–1010.
- Schulz, V., Hänsel, R., & Tyler, V. E. (2001). *Rational phytotherapy* (4th ed.). Springer.
- Sharma, H., & Clark, C. (2012). *Contemporary Ayurveda*. Churchill Livingstone.
- Singh, R. H. (2007). An overview of Ayurveda research. *Ayurveda Journal of Research, 28*(3), 1–10.
- Smith, T., et al. (2019). Clinical efficacy of elderberry in influenza treatment. *Nutrients, 11*(2), 452.
- Stansbury, J. (2018). *Herbal formulas for health practitioners*. Bastyr University Press.
- Tilburt, J. C., & Kaptchuk, T. J. (2008). Herbal medicine research and global health. *World Health Organization Bulletin, 86*(8), 594–599.
- Tindle, H. A., et al. (2005). Trends in use of herbal medicine in the United States. *JAMA, 293*(13), 1569–1576.
- Upton, R. (Ed.). (2011). *American Herbal Pharmacopoeia: Botanical monographs*. American Herbal Pharmacopoeia.
- van Breemen, R. B., & Fong, H. H. (2008). Ensuring quality control of herbal medicines. *Journal of AOAC International, 91*(5), 1304–1308.
- Wachtel-Galor, S., & Benzie, I. F. (2011). *Herbal medicine: Biomolecular and clinical aspects* (2nd ed.). CRC Press.
- Weiss, R. F. (2001). *Herbal medicine* (2nd ed.). Thieme.
- Werner, M., et al. (2019). The role of adaptogens in fatigue management: A systematic review. *Nutrients, 11*(6), 1309.
- World Health Organization. (2013). *WHO traditional medicine strategy 2014–2023*. WHO Press.
- World Health Organization. (2010). *Monographs on selected medicinal plants* (Vols. 1–4). WHO Press.
- Yamada, K., et al. (2011). Anti-allergic properties of nettle leaf extract. *Planta Medica, 77*(13), 1440–1445.
- Zhou, Y., et al. (2018). Anti-inflammatory effects of hibiscus. *Journal of Ethnopharmacology, 213*, 68–78.

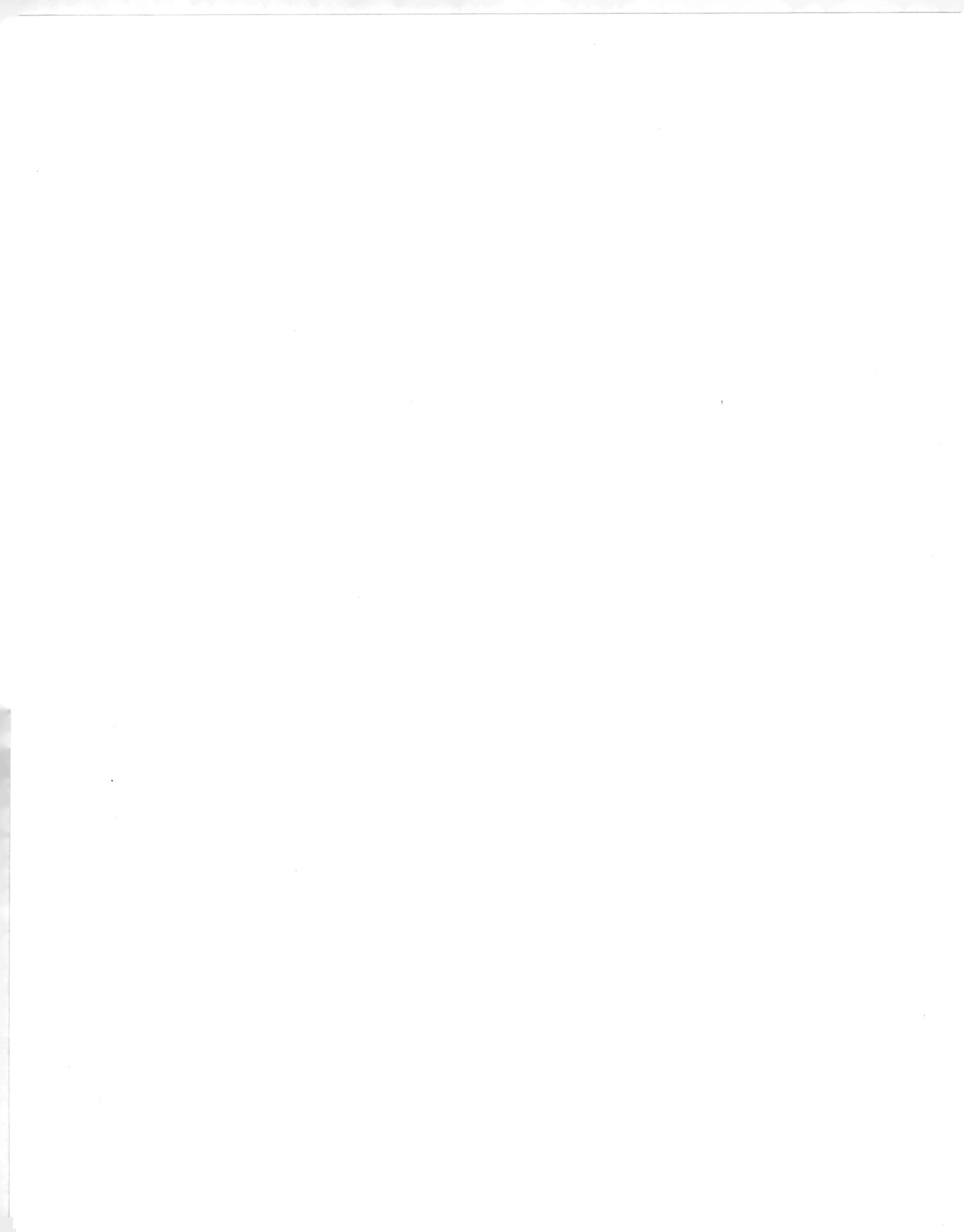